MEDICAL NURSING

NURSES' AIDS SERIES

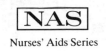

Nurses' Aids Series

MEDICAL NURSING

A Concise Nursing Text

Eleventh Edition

Clive Andrewes
RGN, RMN, BSc (Hons) (Lond.), Dip N (Lond.), RNT
*Senior Lecturer, Princess Alexandra and
Newham College of Nursing and Midwifery, London*

Joyce Smith
RGN, RM, ONC, RCNT, Dip N (Lond.)
*Lecturer, Princess Alexandra and
Newham College of Nursing and Midwifery, London*

BAILLIERE TINDALL
London Philadelphia Toronto Sydney Tokyo

<u>Baillière Tindall</u> 24–28 Oval Road,
W. B. Saunders London NW1 7DX

The Curtis Center,
Independence Square West,
Philadelphia, PA 19106–3399, USA

55 Horner Avenue,
Toronto, Ontario M8Z 4X6, Canada

Harcourt Brace & Company, Australia
32–52 Smidmore Street,
Marrickville, NSW 2204, Australia

Harcourt Brace & Company, Japan
Ichibancho Central Building, 22–1 Ichibancho,
Chiyoda-ku, Tokyo, 102, Japan

© 1992 Baillière Tindall

First published 1941
Tenth edition 1984
Eleventh edition 1992
Third printing 1997

Margaret Hitch wrote the first edition of *Medical Nursing* and
subsequent editions were prepared by Marjorie Houghton, the seventh
in collaboration with Mary Whittow. The eighth and ninth were prepared
by Christine M. Chapman. The tenth edition was written by Gillian M.
Newton and Clive Andrewes.

Typeset by Best-set Typesetter Ltd., Hong Kong
Printed and bound in Great Britain by
Mackays of Chatham PLC, Chatham, Kent

ISBN 0 7020 1454 0

A catalogue record for this book is available from the British Library.

Contents

Preface

It is seven years since this book was last revised. In this period nursing has continued to experience considerable change. Degrees and Diploma-based education continue to develop, reflecting the deepening knowledge base of nursing, with its own theories and research.

Within this framework of change we see the purpose of this book as introducing students, and those returning to nursing, to an understanding of the knowledge, skills and values required to nurse people. This book is only an introduction, and we hope that it will stimulate the reader to explore the subject areas more deeply. In order to facilitate this, further reading lists are suggested at the end of each chapter.

In rewriting this book we have included three new chapters—on nursing, on caring for people with an infection and on caring for people with cancer. We hope this reflects the continuing move of nursing away from the dominance of the medical model, to an area of practice and study in its own right. In addition, we have used a problem-orientated approach to the care people require in the relevant chapters. Goals/aims for problems are not generally stated, as these should be planned in relation to the individual for whom the nurse is caring.

We hope that this book will be of benefit in developing the reader's knowledge, interest and enthusiasm for nursing and encourage them to further their learning about caring for people.

Joyce Smith
Clive Andrewes

Acknowledgements

This book has had an odd hiccough or two from conception to delivery. We would like to thank those sensitive midwives—Sarah Smith and Gill Robinson—at Baillière Tindall for their patience, kindness, support and the appropriate prodding that was required.

We are also grateful to Michael Marek and Natasha Bunford in the College of Nursing and Midwifery, for their help, tolerance and weary sighs over our fledgling word processing skills. Without their help, our panic over information technology would have reached epidemic proportions.

Furthermore, we would like to thank our Principal—Edith Parker—at the Princess Alexandra and Newham College of Nursing and Midwifery. Edith has created an educational environment which encourages students and lecturers to take responsibility for their own learning and development. This philosophy has helped us take on the challenge of writing this book. We promise that we did do it in our own time.

We would also like to thank our busy sisters/charge nurses at The Royal London Hospital Trust, who in the midst of patient care, budgets, and trusts, took time to read selected chapters and help point us in the right direction.

Lastly, we thank our students for their tolerance of our periods of distraction. We are still somewhat unsure what they meant when they said that they had not noticed any difference!

1 Nursing

Most nurses have their own ideas about what nursing is, or
should be. Our beliefs may be based on a private image
of nursing which was shaped by our experiences. This
experience will have been influenced by the portrayal of
nursing through literature and the media.

At the heart of this image often lies the concept of
caring. Nurse theorists have identified caring as a para-
digm unique to nursing. It has been described as the 'core'
or 'essence' of nursing. Despite this recognition that
caring is at the centre of nursing, little agreement exists
about a definition of nursing. Perhaps this is not surprising
when one considers the many different settings within
which nursing is carried out.

Nurses work within both hospital and community
environments. In both these settings nursing may be very
different. The nursing undertaken by a district nurse may
have little in common with that done by a nurse working
in an operating theatre. Even within the same setting
nurses may seem to have very different roles. A nurse
practising as a school nurse may have a different orientation from a nurse who is working for an occupational
health department of a large firm.

At present there are four different registrations that
nurses can obtain at completion of their education/
training. They can become registered general nurses,
registered mental nurses, registered sick children's nurses
or registered nurses in caring for people with learning

difficulties. Recent changes in nurse education mean that for 18 months of their education all nurses now have the same common core of knowledge, before branching out to a particular registration.

In each of these registrations a nurse can, and will now be required to, continue their education. Further specialist qualifications can be obtained. Given the many different ways a nurse can practise, and the difficulty in arriving at an agreed definition of nursing, what knowledge, values and skills do we require as nurses?

In the past, the knowledge and skills required were determined by nurses working within a framework of medical care. What we learnt and the skills we developed were in relation to caring for ill people in hospital settings under the direction of medical staff. Over recent years we have perhaps expanded the sources of knowledge that we feel we need to understand. An understanding of physiology, psychology and sociology has come to be seen as an important part of the theoretical base that the nurse needs to practise nursing.

The last 20 years have seen a further shift. Nurses have now begun to develop their own theories and views, and so a body of knowledge about nursing in its own right has grown up. The reasons for this are varied. They concern, firstly, the desire, if we are to be a profession, to have our own body of knowledge. Secondly, there has been a move to consider the primary role of nursing as being a concern with health and wellness, rather than illness and ill-health.

Thirdly, and of equal importance, there has been the development of individual patient or client care. This has involved nurses separately assessing those they care for, identifying their problems from a nursing perspective, setting outcomes for those problems, planning the care required to alleviate the problems and then evaluating the effectiveness of the care that has been given.

If we are to carry this out, it has been argued that we need frameworks, or maps, to guide our nursing. These maps need not be the same, although they relate to the same area. If one considers a city, then for that same city, a number of different maps can exist. One could have a map of the bus routes, or the streets, or the leisure facilities within that town. The map that you choose to use is determined by what information or guidance you need.

As has been stated, nursing is carried out in many different ways and in varied settings by nurses, so we may need different maps of nursing according to the direction in which we wish to go and the information we feel we need. These maps are referred to as nursing models.

NURSING MODELS

These frameworks, or maps, within which we can organize and deliver individual care to the people we nurse are varied. However, if they are all concerned with nursing, then there should be some common structure to these frameworks. Nursing models should address four main areas. They should have a view of a person, a view of the environment, explain how they see health and ill-health and state how individualized nursing care should be practised. These should not be four separate areas, but need to be linked together, so that the framework we are using is logical.

The person

A nursing model should state a view of what makes a person function and behave the way that they do. What physical needs do we have? What psychological/emotional needs do we have? What spiritual needs do we have? How does a person behave and what motivates them as a result of these needs?

This view of how a person normally functions is critical, as it is the basis on which a nurse must then assess an individual. It is this assessment of how a person's health is normally that enables us to look at the areas which are a problem due to ill-health.

The environment

A nursing model should state a view of how the environment we live in affects an individual. The environment can be physical, e.g. housing, employment and education. It can also concern a person's psycho-social environment, e.g. how does the family unit—of which there are several types—make a difference to how the individual functions?

Health and ill-health

Given the view on how a person functions and how they relate to the environment, the model should then discuss what makes a person healthy and what causes this state of health to be altered.

Health and ill-health can be maintained by a series of factors. These can be physical or psychological or social factors, or a combination of all three. The model should also address the question of who decides when someone is well or unwell.

Nursing

Given that a model has stated how it sees a person, the environment and its effect on an individual and what is meant by wellness and illness, it must then address how individualized nursing should be practised.

INDIVIDUALIZED NURSING CARE

This approach involves a number of stages:

1. Assess the condition of the person being nursed.
2. Identify, from the assessment made, the person's problems.
3. Establish goals or aims in relation to each problem.
4. Plan nursing actions in relation to each problem identified.
5. Carry out the actions decided upon.
6. Evaluate whether the care being given is relieving the problem.

These stages are sometimes summarized into four:

Assessment
Planning
Implementation
Evaluation

These stages are not static. As care is evaluated it is reassessed and the goals and nursing actions may be altered. It is a continuous process (see Figure 1.1).

Nursing care planning has been defined as the 'systematic assessment and identification of problems, the setting of objectives and the establishment of methods and strategies for accompanying them' (Mayers).

Assessment

As part of a person's admission to hospital (see Chapter 2) the nurse must assess the person in order to plan their care. There are a number of sources of information:

- The person themselves.
- Their family.

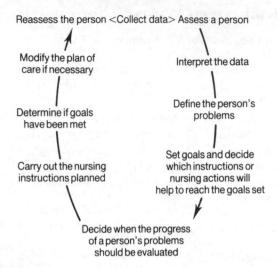

Figure 1.1 Cyclical stages of individualized nursing care.

- A physical screening by the nurse.
- Their medical case notes.

Information about a person is often obtained using a questionnaire-type form. In some instances this information is directly recorded onto a computer screen, as the nursing care plan and progress notes are also computerized.

The first part of this form contains general administrative information. It also includes a section on the care the person has in the community. This should mean that planning the needs and education a person has on returning home should start from admission. An example of a typical front part of this questionnaire is shown in Figure 1.2.

The second part of the assessment form will be designed within the framework of the nursing model that is

NURSING HISTORY

PATIENT PERSONAL DETAILS	MEDICAL PROFILE	COMMUNITY CARE/DISCHARGE PLAN
Name Address	Consultant House Officer Diagnosis	CARE AT HOME Details/Name Community Nurse Social Worker Social Services (Please specify)
Record No. Age Date of birth Time Date of Admission Waiting List Type: Emergency Transfer from Marital Status Religion Next of Kin (name) Relationship to Patient Address	Operations on present admission/date performed Past medical history/operations	G.P. Name Address DISCHARGE PLAN (related health education developed in care plan) Date of Discharge/Transfer Next of Kin/Warden informed Discharge to:
Tel. No(s) Housing: (any problems pertinent to the patient's condition)	Allergies History of present complaint Other current health problems	Community Nurse Social Worker Social Services i.e. Home Help Meals on Wheels Day centre attendance Any Other?
Visiting Problems? Does next of kin know of admission: Yes/No Patient requests no information to be given Informed (who) by at hrs. on ...../...../.9..... WARD	Information about patients condition Given to by date	Medication Out-patients appt. Transport

	Tick if required	Date ordered	Initials of nurse

Figure 1.2 Front sheet of nursing assessment.

used to guide and direct nursing care. Different models put different emphases on the needs and requirements of a person. These will be reflected in the categories that a nurse must use to assess the person who has been admitted.

In order to do this the nurse must have knowledge and understanding of what the particular theorist meant by the categories within the form. An example of this is the category within a model which the authors term dying. Without an understanding of what they mean by this category inappropriate or insensitive questions may be asked.

Two popular frameworks or models used in the United Kingdom are Roper, Tierney and Logan's Activities of Daily Living approach and Dorothea Orem's Self-Care Model of Nursing. Examples of assessment forms which reflect these two approaches are shown in Figures 1.3 and 1.4.

In addition to understanding what the nurse theorist meant by the terms within their approach, the nurse must ensure that the person being assessed understands that this information is required in order to plan their care individually. It is the critical phase of planning individual care. Unless the assessment is carried out skilfully, problems will not be identified and care will be planned inadequately.

The nurse needs both verbal and non-verbal skills to assess a person well. Language must be clear and understood by the person, questions asked with sensitivity and confidentiality and privacy maintained. The same nurse who assesses a person should then plan the care that is required. Ideally, they should then be involved in participating in the delivery and evaluation of that care.

As part of assessing a person's problems the nurse will carry out a physical screening of the person to identify any

ASSESSMENT OF ACTIVITIES OF LIVING

NAME:

T. P. R. BP. W.T.
URINALYSIS

IN EACH ACTIVITY OF LIVING INCLUDE:–
USUAL ROUTINES
WHAT HE/SHE CAN AND CANNOT
DO INDEPENDENTLY

PATIENTS' PROBLEMS
(ACTUAL/POTENTIAL)
(P) – POTENTIAL

MAINTAINING A SAFE ENVIRONMENT	CONTROLLING BODY TEMPERATURE	
COMMUNICATING	MOBILIZING	
BREATHING	WORKING AND PLAYING	
EATING AND DRINKING	EXPRESSING SEXUALITY	
ELIMINATING	SLEEPING/COMFORT	
PERSONAL CLEANSING AND DRESSING	DYING	

DETAILS TAKEN BY: GRADE: DATE:

Figure 1.3 Roper, Tierney and Logan's Activity of Daily Living assessment categories.

SELF-CARE ASSESSMENT

NAME:

T.   P.   R.   BP.   WT.

URINALYSIS

To include:
The demands on the patient's ability to self-care, and the
ability of the patient to meet those demands on self-care.

AIR	SOLITUDE AND SOCIAL INTERACTION
WATER AND FOOD	HAZARDS TO WELL-BEING
SPECIAL SENSES	EFFECTS OF DISEASE
ELIMINATION	EFFECTS OF TREATMENT
ACTIVITY AND REST	

DETAILS TAKEN BY: GRADE: DATE:

Figure 1.4 Orem's Self-Care assessment categories.

actual or potential problems. Blood pressure, cardiac rate, respirations, temperature, urinalysis and the weight of the person will all be assessed.

Identifying problems

Once an assessment has been made the person's problems can be identified. These may be actual or real problems occurring at present, or potential problems that may occur later. Problems should be identified that are relevant to the person's own health. In setting out the problems on a plan of care the priorities of problems should be determined. Problems should be set out according to whether they are:

- Problems that are a threat to life.
- Problems that are currently occurring.
- Possible problems which may occur in the future if something is not done to prevent them.

Setting goals or outcomes for each problem

When each problem is determined, then an outcome for each of the problems should be set. Setting goals is often the area that causes most difficulty. If we are to evaluate whether the problem is resolving then we need a clear goal that can be measured, so goals must be specific and understood in the same way by all members of the nursing team.

Goals such as 'not to be breathless' or 'to feel better' are inadequate, as they are open to different interpretations. A goal such as 'respirations to be below 18 a minute after walking to the lavatory' is clear and could be measured in the same way by nurses. Goals must be written with, or by, the person who is unwell. It is their health and they should determine their own goal for each of the problems identified. If that goal is unrealistic, then the nurse should discuss with the individual why it is unrealistic and the setting of an achievable goal.

For each problem and goal the nurse must then decide on when they should review or evaluate the effectiveness of the care that is being given for each problem.

Nursing actions

Nursing actions related to each problem should be stated. These should be specific, precise and clearly understood in the same way by all the nurses involved in caring for the person. Examples of general instructions which give rise to different interpretations by nurses are 'Encourage or push fluids' and 'Gentle or gradual mobilization'. Communication, and therefore the correct implementation of instructions, is helped if these imprecise phrases are not used. It would be clearer if, for example, for a problem of an inadequate fluid intake with a goal of 2500 ml over 24 hours, the instructions stated: 800 ml between 08.00 and 14.00; 1200 ml between 14.00 and 22.00; and 500 ml between 22.00 and 08.00.

The guidelines for writing instructions or nursing actions are:

- Instructions should be feasible. It must be realistic to perform the care that is planned.
- The instructions should be specific so that no matter which nurse is carrying them out, the interpretation of that instruction will be the same.
- The instruction should relate to a specific problem and goal.
- The person on whom those instructions are to be carried out should understand the reason for the particular nursing action.

An example of a care plan is shown in Figure 1.5.

PATIENT CARE DOCUMENTATION

DATE	NO.	PATIENT PROBLEM/ NEED	GOAL/OUTCOME FOR PATIENT	ACTION	EVALUATION DATE	SIGNATURE	PROBLEM RESOLVED

NAME: AGE: HOSPITAL NO:

Figure 1.5 Example of a care plan.

Implementation of nursing care

There are two main ways that nursing care is being organized: within systems of team nursing and primary nursing. For further information on these two types of approaches to delivering nursing care, see Further reading list.

The principle behind these ways of nursing is that the same nurse should be responsible for assessing a person, working with that person in drawing up the plan of care, carrying out that care and then assessing or evaluating the effectiveness of that care. As the same individual nurse cannot be on duty for the whole time, other nurses must also be involved in the delivery of that care. Therefore the role of the main nurse identified as responsible for caring for an individual, is to be accountable for the organization, implementation and evaluation of the care. Day to day changes can obviously be made by a nurse involved in the care, but the overall plan of care remains the responsibility of the designated nurse.

The care that has been given is recorded on the person's progress notes. An example of a form of progress notes is seen in Figure 1.6. Comments on the progress of a person's care should be written in relation to the problems in the care plan.

Thus, a plan of care has an assessment sheet, a care plan and a form to record the progress of the care that has been given. These latter two forms are sometimes combined as one.

Evaluation

In order to determine if the nursing care that has been given is effective, it must be evaluated. This is a continuous process. It has three main functions:

Figure 1.6 An example of a type of progress note form

DATE REQUESTED	ACTION BY OTHER TEAM MEMBERS/INVESTIGATIONS	DATE COMPLETED	DATE	NO	PROGRESS/EVALUATION	SIGNED

NAME: AGE: HOSPITAL NO:

- To determine whether goals have been met.
- To provide information so that we can reassess a person's needs.
- To determine which nursing actions were effective in a given situation.

Evaluation is critical for the nursing as a whole. It provides information that enables nurses to assess the effectiveness of their care. Nursing actions that fail can be discarded and new approaches planned. Different approaches to the same problem can be evaluated. A body of written information is thus being collected that enables nurses themselves to monitor and assess nursing actions. The information within care plans, whether in written form or on computer disks, can be used as a basis to assess the quality of the nursing care that has been given.

Involvement of the person in planning individual care

The philosophy of beliefs that a group of nurses has will determine not only which nursing framework, or model, they choose to use, but also the role of the person they are caring for in the care they are receiving. Nurses can involve the person in setting out problems and goals for the care they require. The plan of care can be kept at the end of the bed or by a person's locker, or it may be kept on a ward desk or in the office. People can either see and participate in the writing of their own progress notes, or this can remain the prerogative of the nursing staff.

This system or approach to care allows nurses to involve the people they are caring for in the way they believe. There is no right or wrong way, as long as individual nurses are accountable for, and are therefore prepared to justify, the way that they are nursing and how they are involving the person whom that nursing is designed to help.

These different approaches mean that nurses must agree, within one area of practice, on a consistent approach. If we are not using the same map we will all go off in different directions! The main reasons for using a model are well summarized by Alan Pearson and Barbara Vaughan (1986):

'If a team of nurses agree to base their practice on a generally accepted model, it will:

1. Lead to consistency to the sort of care received by patients and thus to a continuity of care patterns and treatment.
2. Give rise to less conflict within the team of nurses as a whole.
3. Make sense of the nursing given by the team; the other health care workers involved, such as doctors, physiotherapists and social workers will understand the logic behind the care.
4. Give direction to nursing care within the area, since the goals of nursing work will be understood by the whole team.
5. Act as a major guide in decision and policy making because the components of the model chosen can act as a guide against which to check decisions.
6. Act as a guide for the criteria on which new team members are selected.'

Choosing a model to direct our nursing can be difficult. A variety of models exist with different views of a person, the environment, health, ill-health and nursing. In more instances now, nurses are designing, or creating, their own model of care, based on their own expertise and the area in which they nurse.

Whichever framework is chosen, or designed, it should reflect the elements within Riehl and Roy's definition of a nursing model; a

'systematically constructed, scientifically based and logically related set of concepts which identify the essential components of nursing practice together with the theoretical bases for these concepts and the values required in their use by the practitioner.'

FURTHER READING

AGGLETON, P. & CHALMERS, H. (1984). Models and theories: defining the terms. *Nursing Times*, **80**(36), 24–28.

CHAPMAN, C. (1985). *Theory of Nursing: Practical Application*. Harper and Row, London.

FITZPATRICK, J. J. & WHALL, A. L. (1983). *Conceptual Models of Nursing*. F. A. Davies and Company, Philadelphia.

HUNT, J. & MARKS-MARRAN, D. (1980). *Nursing Care Plans—The Nursing Process at Work*. HM & M Publications, London.

MARRINER, A. (1983). *The Nursing Process*, 3rd edn. C.V. Mosby, St Louis.

MARRINER, A. (1986). *Nursing Theorists and their Work*. C.V. Mosby, St Louis.

McFARLANE, J. & CASTLEDINE, G. (1982). *The Practice of Nursing using the Nursing Process*. C.V. Mosby, London.

OREM, D. (1980). *Nursing Concepts of Practice*, 2nd edn. McGraw Hill, New York.

PEARSON, A. & VAUGHAN, B. (1986). *Nursing Model for Practice*. Heinemann, London.

RIEHL, J. P. & ROY, C. (1984). *Conceptual Models for Nursing Practice*, 3rd edn. Appleton-Century Croft, Norwalk.

ROPER, N., LOGAN, W. & TIERNEY, L. (1985). *The Elements of Nursing*, 2nd edn. Churchill Livingstone, Edinburgh.

ROPER, N. (1990). *Using a Model of Nursing*, 5th edn. Churchill Livingstone, Edinburgh.

ROY, C. (1976). *Introduction to Nursing: an Adaptation Model*. Prentice Hall, Englewood Cliffs, New Jersey.

STEVENS, B. J. (1979). *Nursing Theory: Analysis, Application, Evaluation*. Little Brown, Boston.

WRIGHT, S. G. (1986). *Building and Using a Model of Nursing*. Edward Arnold, London.

2   People in hospital

Admission to hospital is a stressful experience. The person facing hospital is anxious over their health, what is going to happen to them, their family and life outside hospital and the strange environment they are entering. These worries become more complex as they are transformed by the admission procedure from a person into a patient. Their life outside hospital and their individuality diminish as they assume their role in the institution of a hospital. Nurses have a critical role in reducing the effects of this process of depersonalization.

ADMISSION TO HOSPITAL

People are normally admitted in a planned way from home or as an emergency through the casualty department. They enter a ward dressed in their own clothes. They may be accompanied by relatives or friends, who are often asked to wait outside the ward. They are taken to their bed, the curtains are drawn and they are asked to undress. They put on their nightwear, place their clothes in a locker and then often get into bed or sit in a chair by the bed. An identity band is placed around their wrist. Their family say goodbye and go home. They have now become a patient in a numbered bed.

In many cases this transformation need not be so rapid and bleak. The process of admission should be organized so as to prevent dehumanization and help a person retain their individuality. There are a number of ways in which this can be done:

- There is often little point in undressing so quickly, as the doctor's examination may not take place for several hours. In addition, there may be no reason why people should not wear their own clothes for the greater part of their admission. This can help them to feel like an individual and not a cog in a machine.

- People and their families should be warmly welcomed to the ward and shown where the day room and lavatories are. The different grades of nurses and how the nursing is organized within the ward should be explained. A drink should be offered, as they may have travelled some distance or had a long wait before coming to the ward.

- Physical screening by nurses, assessing blood pressure, temperature, cardiac and respiratory rate, weight and urinalysis should be carried out as part of the nursing assessment. There can be a tendency for these aspects of nursing to be carried out immediately on admission. If this happens, it can only strengthen the person's feeling of being on an assembly line.

- The aim should be that admission should be calm, friendly and unhurried. Anxiety should be reduced by providing information and ensuring that the person feels that they are valued as an individual.

It is worth reflecting on the extent to which we, as nurses, and the person being admitted, feel the need to create a 'patient role'. When roles are well established, both nurse and patient know their place and may feel secure and safe. The creation of such a structured relationship may make it easier for the nurses to give, and the patient to receive, physical nursing care. However, the cost may be that the psychological and emotional care that is required may be inadequate, and so recovery and healing may be delayed.

The aim of the nurse should be to care for the person as a whole. If individuality is reduced, this approach cannot be fulfilled. The person will become the 'patient in bed ten with a heart attack'. As the process of admission is the introduction to nursing for the person, it is important that this process emphasizes, rather than diminishes, the person's feeling that they as an individual person are important.

The process of admission, during which assessment of the person, so as to plan individual nursing care, is carried out, should be organized in order to:

- Introduce the relationship between the nurse and the person who is unwell.
- Strengthen the nurse's perception of the person as an individual.
- Help the person understand and feel that they will be cared for as an individual, with a family and life outside hospital.

CARING FOR A PERSON IN HOSPITAL

A person admitted to hospital will cope with the stress they undergo as they cope with other stresses in their lives. They will have learnt ways to buffer themselves against anxiety and external dangers. These defence mechanisms, such as repression, reaction formation, rationalization, insulation and projection, are designed for self-protection. They enable us to cope with our environment.

In hospital, a person is subjected to many different stresses. Their ability to manage their anxiety may be tested to its limits. People are concerned about their ill-health, their family and their new environment. In addition, they are subject to a series of fears about tests they are undergoing, operations that may be required, how well they will become and a series of issues related to life in hospital.

One of the major ways that nurses can help relieve these feelings and demonstrate caring, which is at the heart of the nurse–patient interaction, is through communication. Communication is essential for the establishment and maintenance of human relationships. It is the way that people in hospital obtain information about themselves, share feelings and thoughts with nurses about their ill-health, keep in contact with their families and relate to other people within a ward environment.

Communication is carried out both verbally and non-verbally, or, as it is sometimes expressed, talking with or without words.

Verbal communication

Use of language involves the skills of:

- Speaking
- Listening
- Reading and writing

Speaking involves not only what is said, but also how it is said. Messages about feeling are conveyed by the tone and inflection of the voice. 'Would you like another cup of tea?' can be asked in a friendly, positive way or in a grudging, negative manner.

When information is given, it should be precise and free of nursing or medical jargon. It is often helpful if the nurse asks the person to report back, in their own words, what they have said. This ensures they understand what was meant by the explanation.

In our multi-racial society some people may not speak English. In this case, a relative or interpreter can be used to convey information to them, and non-verbal communication assumes great importance.

Listening is an active process; it is much more than just hearing. It involves sharing information and feelings. Encouraging the person to express themselves will not be helped if the person senses you are not listening. It means being attentive, not being silent.

Reading and writing are skills which are often taken for granted. There are, however, a large number of people who are unable to perform these skills and to assume that they can may cause distress and embarrassment.

Non-verbal communication/talking without words

Non-verbal communication can be the most effective means a nurse has of allaying fears and anxieties. It is a two-way method of communication that involves our five senses. Actions are transmitted as clearly as the spoken word, and they are understood as readily. Some actions communicate messages; others convey information about feelings or personality.

Body language

Gestures, movements of the body, facial expressions and posture all communicate messages. The way one approaches a person is vital in establishing a relationship. A smile, eye contact and an open posture, suggest friendliness and interest. The posture of a person who is huddled up in bed, with their back to the nurse, suggests withdrawal, apathy or depression. An illustration of how body language can convey information is shown in Figure 2.1.

A nurse needs to be aware of the messages being given by their own body, and those being sent by the individual in hospital.

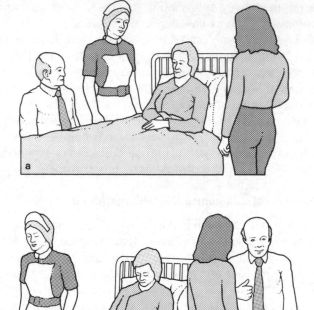

Figure 2.1 Examples of (a) good communication, and (b) poor communication using body language.

Touch

In nursing, touch may be the most important of all non-verbal behaviours. It is the most personal of our senses as it brings two human beings into a direct relationship. It is through touch that we feel the emotions of others. It is clearly a very powerful method of communication.

People are touched by nurses continually. It is an

integral part of most nursing procedures. How the nurse
handles or touches a person says a great deal about the
way they feel about them and their illness. Similarly,
touch tells the nurse a lot about a person's physical and
emotional condition. Resting a hand on someone's
shoulder, or holding their hand, can provide more emotional support than any number of words. Recognition
of the importance of touch has perhaps diminished in
modern medicine and nursing. However, its role should
always be remembered.

Other aspects of non-verbal communication include
periods of silence, the concept of territory, time, and
vocalization (i.e. all aspects of sound—pitch, tone,
screams, gasps, sighs, etc.).

Anxiety and stress are part of a person's life in hospital.
Through verbal and non-verbal communication, the nurse
must understand and meet the needs of the people being
nursed. Therefore an understanding of the methods of
communication is essential, or fears and worries will be
ignored. Instead of nursing the person as a whole, only the
physical problems will be cared for.

Meeting a person's needs in a constructive way will not
only help them during their period in hospital, but will
also enable them to re-enter their environment outside
hospital more easily.

DISCHARGE FROM HOSPITAL

Discharge from hospital is usually seen as a pleasant
event. However, for some people it can be accompanied
by stress. Many people are discharged on the same day as
they are told they can go home. Anxieties can arise about
the journey home, coping on arriving there, and the
sudden change of environment. In addition, there are

worries over drugs, possible dietary restrictions, and what activities should or should not be carried out.

The nurse has an important role in planning the person's discharge so as to ease these concerns, acting as a co-ordinator of the people who are to give advice and arrange help in the community.

Throughout a person's stay in hospital, care should be given while bearing in mind the person's family and home environment. They should not be nursed solely within the framework of the hospital. The assessment of the person on admission and during their stay in hospital should reveal needs associated with the home situation. There are a number of factors of particular importance.

Need for understanding about the illness and its consequences

Advice and understanding about a person's illness is often necessary for the individual and their family, if health is to be maintained.

- Knowledge about drugs regularly required and their side-effects is essential. Where possible, people should have their own drugs before discharge. They are then able to take them under supervision, and can familiarize themselves with when to take them and in what doses.
- Advice about diet may be required. The dietician should see the person and their family before discharge and, if possible, a person should choose their own diet on the ward. It is of little benefit if their diet is given to them the moment before they go home, as they will have had no practice at choosing the correct foods.
- Information about the range and extent of activities which can be undertaken is often required. There may be restrictions on the amount of exercise, and on when

to return to work or to resume sexual relationships. There are explanatory leaflets on many diseases which may be helpful, e.g. *A Heart Attack*, which is one of a series of booklets published by the British Heart Foundation.

- Information about the disease itself may be necessary. A person may need to recognize when they are having a hypo- or hyperglycaemic attack, or may need to know what to do if they are getting chest pain.

Ability to be independent

A person's ability to manage when they go home must be considered in advance of their discharge. There are a number of services and aids which can be of help.

- A person may have nursing needs when at home. They may be unable to give their own insulin injection, or may need a nurse to perform a wound dressing. Community nurses can be arranged to help with such problems.
- They may be unable to shop, cook or look after their own house, and thus home helps or meals-on-wheels may need to be arranged.
- A home assessment by the occupational therapist and social worker may be undertaken. If required, practical aids such as a commode, rails in the bathroom, or a different bed can be arranged.

Living accommodation

Practical aids can help make a person's accommodation suitable for their discharge from hospital. In certain cases, the type of accommodation itself will need to be assessed.

A person may be unable to manage stairs, may now be in a wheelchair, or may have a degree of physical disability which makes managing in the original environment impracticable. Much may depend on the amount of family support that is available. If necessary, alternative arrangements can be made: new housing, a sheltered flat or a local authority home can all be considered.

Follow-up care

It is important for a person to know how their future care is to be arranged. Their level of health may need to be observed and their treatment may need to be altered. General practitioners must be informed about discharge and treatment while the person is still in hospital. An out-patient appointment may be given. Unless appropriate follow-up care is organized, ill-health may return.

The above factors should all be considered when a person is discharged from hospital. They should be remembered throughout the admission, so that planning a person's discharge occurs at the beginning of their stay in hospital. Care will be of limited benefit unless people and their problems are related to their environment outside hospital.

CONCLUSION

In caring for people in hospital the nurse must consider them as individuals with families and lives outside the hospital walls. It is all too easy in a busy ward environment for a person to become just a patient in bed with a disease.

Individuality must be maintained by ensuring that the process of admission to hospital, caring while in hospital and preparing a person to return home are integrated actions. Admission and assessment should heighten and strengthen the perception of the person that they are an individual, by the skilled and sensitive way in which it is organized. Part of that process is thinking about the person's needs on admission, in relation to the time when they will go home.

We must remember that each person is an individual and not label them as a patient with all the stigma that can be attached to that dehumanizing term.

FURTHER READING

ARGYLE, M. (1983). *The Psychology of Interpersonal Behaviour*, 4th edn. Penguin, London.

BREARLEY, S. (1990). *Patient Participation*. Scutarri Press, Harrow, London.

BRIDGE, W. & MACLEOD CLARK, J. (1981). *Communication in Nursing Care*. Wiley, Chichester.

GOFFMAN, E. (1961). *Asylums—Essays in the Social Situation of Mental Patients and Other Inmates*. Penguin, London.

GOFFMAN, E. (1963). *Stigma*. Penguin, London.

PEPLAU, H. E. (1981). *Interpersonal Relations in Nursing*. MacMillan Education, London.

ROBERTS, I. (1975). *Discharged from Hospital*. Royal College of Nursing, London.

SCHNEIDER, D. J., HESTORF, A. H. & ELLSWORTH, P. E. (1970). *Person Perception*. Addison Wesley, London.

SIMPSON, P. J. E. & LEVITT, E. (1981). *Going Home: A Guide For Helping the Patient on Leaving Hospital*. Churchill Livingstone, Edinburgh.

STOCKWELL, F. (1972). *The Unpopular Patient*. Royal College of Nursing, London.

WILSON-BARNETT, J. (ed.) (1983). *Patient Teaching*. Churchill Livingstone, London.

3 Nursing the dependent person

This chapter is concerned with the essential nursing care which may be encountered when nursing the dependent person. Subsequent chapters will give specific guidelines to the nursing care and problems relevant to the area under discussion.

The human body is designed for motion. All internal and external organs must move about to function and these organs are interdependent.

When the activity of the body is greatly decreased, the body functions are directly affected and potential problems for the dependent person can occur.

Using the problem-solving approach allows the nurse to care for the person as an individual: by taking an accurate admission history in which information can be gained on which to base an assessment of the person's problems. The identification of the physical, emotional, spiritual and cultural components of these problems enables the nurse to set realistic aims and deliver the required care and continuously evaluate the effectiveness of this care.

PROBLEMS ASSOCIATED WITH CHANGE OF ENVIRONMENT AND ROUTINE

Depersonalization caused by:

- Unfamiliar ward routine.
- Lack of privacy.

- Lessened decision making.
- Worries about job and family.
- Loss of self-esteem.
- Change in social status from being active and independent to inactive and dependent.

Aim

For the person to feel that they still have control over their life.

Actions

- Give adequate information about care to the person and opportunities to ask questions, so they can make decisions about their own care.
- Involve family/partner and other health professionals, e.g. social worker, physiotherapist, occupational therapist.
- (See Chapter 2)

PROBLEMS ASSOCIATED WITH EATING AND DRINKING

A person's nutritional requirements may be altered during the course of the illness. When fever or infection is present, there is an increased metabolic rate. Toxins suppress the appetite, and if illness is prolonged and nutritional intake inadequate, malnutrition may occur.

Aim

That the person will enjoy and eat a well-balanced diet suitable for their needs, and maintain their normal body weight.

Actions

- Assess reasons why the person may not have the ability or the motivation to eat or drink:
- Assess person for any impairment of manual dexterity, as supportive cutlery may be beneficial.
- Check that the person is comfortable and sitting up and well. This makes eating easier for the person.
- Assess cultural and religious beliefs regarding diet.
- Allow the person as far as possible their choice in food.
- A drink must be easily available.
- Offer foods which stimulate the flow of saliva, e.g. oranges, pineapples.
- If the person is unable to feed themselves the nurse will take the meal to the bedside and take care to sit down by the person, chat to them and try to promote a relaxed and unhurried atmosphere and consult with the person how they like to eat their meals.
- Unless there is any reason not to, most people would prefer to be fed with a fork for their main course.
- Notice the person's reaction to their meal. Are they enjoying it?
- Frequent mouth care
  - Toothbrush and paste for people who can clean their own teeth.
  - For people who are unable to clean their own teeth and mouth, care must be given by the nurse.
  - If the person has dentures, ensure they are clean and comfortable.

During an acute illness, food should be fluid or semi-fluid at first. Milk, eggs, cooked cereals and custards are useful foods in such cases. The fluid intake should be two to three litres a day, unless contraindicated. Later the person may appreciate a light diet such as creamed chicken, fish, pureed vegetables, or stewed fruit.

Vitamin supplements may be necessary if the illness lasts for some time. If bed-rest is prolonged, demineralization of bones may occur because the normal weight-bearing areas are not being used. A good calculation of fluid intake is essential to prevent formation of renal calculi.

Problem

Increase in weight

Aim

That the person will not increase their normal body weight. Some people (e.g. loss of leg function) may overeat and gain excess weight, because their calorie intake is in excess of their diminished energy requirements.

Actions

• Counsel the person about the problems of gaining weight.
• Involve the dietician to give advice.

Drinking

Potential problem

Dehydration can be caused by insufficient fluid intake, loss of fluid by vomiting, excessive urinary output, rapid respirations, and haemorrhage.

Aim

Maintain a fluid balance appropriate for the individual.

Actions

- To provide variety in the types of fluid offered.
- Assess the reasons why the person is not drinking, e.g.
  - Difficulty in reaching and holding cup.
  - Embarrassed and worried because they may wet the bed. (Enssure that commode or bedpan is available.)
  - Record fluid balance (person must be in positive fluid balance).
  - Electrolyte imbalance will occur in severe dehydration and correction will be necessary.
  - Test urine daily—S.G. (Specific Gravity).

Nausea/Vomiting

Nausea and vomiting are common problems. There are a variety of reasons why they may occur.

Predisposing causes

Infection
- food poisoning.
- systemic infection.
Dietary indiscretions, e.g. over-indulgence in alcohol.
Poisons
Drugs, e.g.
- morphine.
- cytotoxic drugs.
Stress
Disorders of the gastrointestinal tract, e.g.
- peptic ulceration.
- obstruction.
- hiatus hernia.
Side-effects of other disorders
- renal failure.
- cardiac failure.

Radiation
Pregnancy

Aim

To alleviate vomiting and nausea.

Actions

- Assist the medical staff in treating the cause.
- Give anti-emetic drugs, e.g.
  - metoclopramide
  - prochlorperazine
  - cyclizine
- Measure fluid intake, loss and vomit.
- Perform mouth care frequently.
- Control pain.
- Alleviate stress.
- Maintain adequate fluid intake.

If the vomiting is prolonged, the person may need intra-venous fluid and electrolyte replacement.

PROBLEMS ASSOCIATED WITH RESPIRATION

Potential problem

Chest infection

Aim

That the person has a clear airway to breath sufficiently well to allow adequate oxygenation of the lungs and tissues.

Actions

- Monitor respiratory rate.
- Encourage deep breathing and coughing.

MEDICAL NURSING

- Supply tissues and sputum pot within reach of the person.
- If condition allows, sit well upright in bed, well supported by pillows. It has been demonstrated that in the upright position the base of the lung is better ventilated.
- Consult physiotherapist for correct breathing exercises and plan nursing care to fit in with this.
- Change person's position frequently.
- Encourage good fluid intake, and high-fibre diet (constipation because of strain and anxiety can cause problems of dyspnoea.)

Education/Support

Explain to the person how important it is to maintain the correct position in bed and to practise their deep breathing exercises.

PROBLEMS ASSOCIATED WITH ELIMINATION

Urinary

Potential problems

- Inactivity may lead to increased deposits of calcium in the renal tract, leading to renal calculi.
- Person may be embarrassed to request bedpans/urinals too often, leading to inadequate emptying of the bladder. The stasis of urine in the bladder will lead to growth of bacteria and bladder infection.

Aim

- To encourage and discuss with the person a plan of care to deal with any problems.

- That the person feels that their dignity is being maintained.

Actions

- Maintain adequate fluid intake unless contraindicated.
- Monitor and record intake and output daily.
- The person, whenever possible, should go out to the toilet to ensure privacy. If this is not possible a commode may be provided and the bed well screened from other people.
- It is essential that the person is able to get to the toilet easily without delay. Some people may have problems with manual dexterity, e.g. rheumatoid arthritis (so it may be necessary to change the fastenings of garments).
- Frequent urine testing is necessary because of the possibility of infection.

Bowels

Potential problems

The lack of exercise, slower blood flow, loss of appetite, pain and drugs can lead to constipation/faecal impaction with overflow diarrhoea.

Aim

To discuss with the person a plan for regular bowel elimination for them based on their normal habits.

Actions

- Adequate fluid intake.
- High-fibre diet. Encourage the person to eat plenty of fruit and vegetables.

- Encourage as much mobility and exercise as the person can manage.
- Check that the person can get a comfortable position either on a commode or in the toilet.
- The provision of privacy, odour-free atmosphere and facilities for personal hygiene are essential.
- Aperients, suppositories or enemas may have to be given. Aperients which are commonly used include faecal softeners such as Mil-Par or liquid paraffin. Bulk purgatives such as methylcellulose or Isogel, or disaccharides such as lactulose Dorbanex senna and bisacodyl (Dulcolax), are also used.

  Glycerine or bisacodyl suppositories may be inserted into the rectum and should be retained for about 20 minutes.
- The most commonly used enema is sodium phosphate, which is supplied in a disposable sachet. This should be inserted high up at the side of the rectum and retained for about 20 minutes.
- Occasionally, retention enemas such as arachis oil may be necessary to soften the faeces.

PROBLEMS ASSOCIATED WITH MOBILITY

Potential problems

Muscle wasting, joint stiffness, overstretching of tendon, e.g. foot drop caused by the inactivity and poor positioning of limbs and joints. Demineralization of bones may also occur because the normal weight-bearing areas are not being used.

Aim

To maintain the normal function and movements of limbs and joints.

Actions

- Encourage active limb exercises or perform passive ones.
- Position and support limbs carefully.

Skin

Potential problem

- Skin breakdown caused by squashing of subcutaneous tissues preventing adequate blood flow.
- The parts of the body susceptible to skin breakdown and the formation of pressure sores are those over the bony prominences, especially the sacral area, hips, heels, elbows.

The effects of this unrelieved pressure will be:

- blistering of the skin
- breaking of the skin
- superficial necrosis and ulcer formation
- gangrene
- sloughing

Predisposing causes

In elderly people
- loss of skin resilience.
- immobility.
- incontinence.
In the paralysed person
- loss of sensation.
- immobility.
- incontinence.
In the oedematous person
- loss of skin resilience.

In the debilitated wasted person
- poor nutrition.
- infections.
- anaemia.
In the unconscious person
- immobility.
- incontinence.
In the person with a splint or any other appliance

In the obese person
- respiration.
- immobility.

- friction.
- immobility.

Aim

For the person's skin to remain intact.

Actions

- All people on admission should be assessed and then reassessed at appropriate intervals, depending on their risk of skin damage.
- An 'at-risk' scoring system such as the Norton Scale or Waterlow Scale can be used to determine which people are particularly susceptible to pressure sores. Examples of two systems of scoring are given in Figures 3.1 and 3.2.
- Turning and repositioning the person two-hourly will allow for normal blood flow.
- When turning the person examine the skin for redness or any other damage.
- Keep the skin clean and dry. Keep the bed free from crumbs and wrinkles.
- Pay attention to food and fluid intake.

PROBLEMS ASSOCIATED WITH PERSONAL CLEANSING AND DRESSING

Potential problem

Difficulty in maintaining personal hygiene.

Aim

To maintain the self-esteem of the person.

Actions

- Give facilities and support for the person to do as much as they can for themself; give help where needed.
- Bathing and attention to skin, hair, teeth and mouth care will promote self-esteem for the person.

PROBLEMS ASSOCIATED WITH PAIN

Problem

Pain is an unpleasant problem which can cause people distress and great discomfort.

Figure 3.1 'At-risk' scoring system for pressure sores. Patients who score a total of 14 or less on this scale are considered to be at risk of developing a pressure sore

	Score			
	1	2	3	4
A. General physical condition	Very bad	Poor	Fair	Good
B. Mental state	Stuporous	Confused	Apathetic	Alert
C. Activity	Bed fast	Chair-bound	Walks with help	Ambulant
D. Mobility	Immobile	Very limited	Slightly limited	Full
E. Incontinence	Double	Usually urinary	Occasionally	Never

From Norton, D., McLaren, R. and Exton-Smith, A. N. (1962) *An Investigation of Geriatric Nursing Problems in Hospital.* With kind permission of the authors and the publishers, The National Corporation for the Care of Old People, London.

Ring scores in table, add total
Several scores per category can be used

Build/weight for height	*	Risk areas visual skin type	*	Sex Age	*
Average	0	Healthy	0	Male	1
above average	1	Tissue paper	1	Female	2
Obese	2	Dry	1	14–49	1
Below average	3	Oedematous	1	50–64	2
		Clammy	1	65–74	3
Continence	*	Discoloured	2	75–80	4
		Broke/spot	3	81 +	5
Complete/Catheterized	0				
Occasion incontinent	1	Mobility	*	Appetite	*
Cath/incontinent of faeces	2	Fully	0	Average	0
Doubly incontinent	3	Restless/Fidgety	1	Poor	1
		Apathetic	2	Nasogastric tube	
		Restricted	3	Fluids only	2
		Inert/traction	4	NBM/Anorexic	3
		Chairbound	5		

Score: 10 + at risk   15 + high risk

Special Risks	*		
Tissue Malnutrition	*	Major surgery/Trauma	*
eg. Terminal cachexia	8	Orthopaedic-	
Cardiac failure	5	below waist, spinal	5
Peripheral vascular		On Table >2 hrs	5
Disease	5		
Anaemia	2	Medication	*
Smoking	1	Steroids, Cytotoxics,	
Neurological Deficit:	*	Anti-inflammatory	4
eg. Diabetes, CVA M.S. Paraplegia; Motor/sensory	4–6	20 + very high risk	

Figure 3.2 The Waterlow risk assessment card. Reproduced from *Nursing Times* (1981) Volume 83 No 39 with permission.

Aim

For the person to feel that the pain is controlled.

Actions

- Assist medical staff in treating the reason for the pain.
- Relieve the anxiety and the stress by explanation.
- Allow the person to express their feelings about the pain.
- Monitor the pain and the effect of analgesia using a pain chart (see Figure 5.2).
- Lift the person correctly.
- Assist the person to attain a comfortable position.
- Apply warmth (or cold) to the affected area.
- Occupy the person's attention by conversation, television, games, where appropriate.
- Give analgesia before pain returns, then adjust the dose down or up to a maintenance level. Common analgesics are:
  Paracetamol or asprin (weak analgesic)
  Codeine or distalgesic (weak narcotics)

Morphine
Diamorphine
Pethidine
Papaveretum ⎬ Narcotic analgesia

- Vomiting is a common side-effect of narcotic analgesia.
- Anti-emetic drugs may be required.
- Achieve comfort by treating other nursing problems such as constipation, dysuria, urinary retention, or breathlessness.
- Alcohol may be given in small quantities.

Surgical procedures such as chordotomies (division of antero-lateral column of the spinal cord) and nerve blocks may be used to relieve pain. Radiotherapy may be used when the cause of pain is malignant disease. Battery-operated stimulators may be used to control some forms of pain.

PROBLEMS ASSOCIATED WITH TEMPERATURE CONTROL

Problem

Pyrexia—a body temperature above 37.2°C.

Predisposing causes

Infection
Inflammation
Dehydration
Excessive heat
Cerebral lesions
Necrosis, e.g. myocardial infarction

Aim

To reduce body temperature to within normal limits or to promote comfort.

Actions

- Assist medical staff in treating the cause.
- Estimate fluid loss through sweating and increase fluid intake accordingly.

- Perform mouth care at least two-hourly.
- Advise the person to wear cotton clothing.
- Advise the person to rest in bed.
- Give a high-protein, high-calorie diet.
- Fan the person if their temperature rises above 38°C.
- Change the sheets frequently.
- Give analgesia for headaches and aching joints—aspirin will relieve pain and reduce temperature.
- Record vital signs and maintain a fluid intake and output chart.
- Reduce body temperature by tepid sponging if it rises above 40.5°C.

A rigor is an attack of severe shivering associated with a rapid rise in temperature. There are three stages:

1. Uncontrollable shivering as the temperature rises rapidly. The person feels cold to touch and has a rapid pulse.
2. Restlessness as the temperature continues to rise. The person feels very hot and thirsty. Their skin is hot and dry. They often complain of headaches.
3. Profuse sweating is followed by a fall in temperature and pulse rate.

The person should be kept warm during the first stage and should be given hot drinks. During the second stage, blankets should be removed and the person should be fanned. Cool drinks are helpful. During the third stage sweat should be wiped from the person's face, neck and chest to prevent discomfort. Bed clothes should be changed. The person's temperature should be recorded every 15 minutes during the rigor. The person will appreciate being washed when the rigor is over.

Problem

Hypothermia—a body temperature below 35°C.

Predisposing causes

Exposure to cold, particularly in the very young and elderly
– lack of heating.
– insufficient clothing.
– insufficient food.
– immobility.
Hypothyroidism (myxoedema), when the body's metabolic rate is reduced
Overdosage of certain drugs, e.g. barbiturates

Aim

To increase body temperature to within normal limits.

Actions

- Assist the medical staff in treating the cause.
- Vital signs and level of consciousness should be monitored. A low-reading rectal thermometer will be necessary to record body temperature. (Rapid rewarming should be avoided as vasodilation will cause the blood pressure to drop and heat loss to increase.)
- Re-warm the person slowly in a warm room.
- Cover the person with an insulating 'space' blanket to preserve heat.
- Give at least three litres of fluid to correct dehydration.

Education/Support

Assess housing situation and the need for socio-economic support. Advise the person on what actions to take to keep warm.

PROBLEMS ASSOCIATED WITH INSOMNIA

Predisposing factors

Stress or anxiety
Discomfort
Depression
Noise
Disturbance, e.g. frequent nursing observations
No apparent cause

Aim

To assist the person to regain a normal sleep pattern.

Actions

- Relieve anxiety by counselling, e.g. listening to problems, explaining procedures.
- Assist the person to achieve a comfortable position.
- Relieve discomfort and control pain.
- Allow the person to assume their normal bedtime habits as assessed from the nursing history where this is possible.
- Give alcohol in small quantities, especially to the elderly.
- Give a hot drink or a small meal at bedtime.
- Assist the person to empty their bladder.
- Give a hypnotic or sedative.

PROBLEMS ASSOCIATED WITH CIRCULATION

Potential problems

Thrombo-embolism
Deep vein thrombosis   } Caused by reduced flow due
Pulmonary embolism   to the inactivity of the person

Deep vein thrombosis

Deep vein thrombosis is a solid clot of blood occurring in
the deep veins of the leg. Forty per cent of such clots are
bilateral. The thrombosis may extend along the full length
of the blood vessel.

Predisposing factors

Predisposing factors to the formation of deep vein thrombosis are:

Stasis

- reduced cardiac output.
- lack of muscular activity.
- varicose veins.
- decreased venous return.

Damage to the vessel wall

- external pressures, e.g. plasters, pillows.
- trauma.
- diseases of the vessel.

Increased viscosity of the blood

- contraceptive pill.
- pregnancy.
- polycythaemia.
- after surgery, due to shock.
- childbirth.

Aim

To prevent these problems occurring.

Actions

- Deep breathing exercises help the venous blood to return to the head.
- Leg exercises utilize the muscular pump to squeeze blood upwards.
- Both these types of exercises should be performed by all people who are at risk of developing a deep vein thrombosis.
- Ideally they should be performed for five minutes of each hour.
- People who are unable to perform these exercises alone should be assisted by nursing staff, physiotherapists and relatives.
- Anti-embolic stockings should be worn by high-risk people. Subcutaneous heparin is sometimes given prophylactically, e.g. prior to surgery.

Assessment

Calf pain—worse on dorsiflexion of the foot (Holman's sign)
Tenderness of the calf
Oedema of calf or foot
Inflammation
Local redness
Increased heat

Medical investigations and treatment

Ultrasound or phlebography may be used in the diagnosis of deep vein thrombosis.

Anticoagulant therapy is started immediately. Drugs are given to slow down the coagulation time of blood. A drug that is commonly used is heparin, which acts rapidly and is used for the first two or three days. It may be given intravenously or subcutaneously.

Warfarin, an oral anticoagulant, takes longer to act. A 'loading' dose is given 24 to 48 hours before the heparin is stopped. Thereafter a daily dose of warfarin is given. Blood is taken daily to determine the prothrombin time ratio (PTR) which indicates how long the blood takes to clot; from this result the dose of warfarin needed is decided.

Actions

- Encourage the person to rest in bed for a few days.
- Elevate the foot of the bed—this will promote venous return—and the use of a bed cradle will relieve the pressure of the bedclothes.
- Advise the person to drink at least two litres of fluid per day; this will help to prevent increased viscosity of the blood.
- Supplement the diet with bran, fruit and vegetables to avoid constipation.
- Encourage the person to do deep breathing exercises.
- After a few days rest the person is allowed to get up and resume normal activities.
- Test the urine daily for blood and observe the person for signs of bruising, as there is a risk of haemorrhage with anticoagulation.

Education/Support

The person will need advice about the frequency of blood tests, the need to carry a card recording their drug, its dose and their blood clotting result and observe for any signs of bleeding/bruising.

Pulmonary embolus

Pulmonary embolus occurs when a portion of thrombus from a systemic vein is detached and enters the circulation. It may lodge in a pulmonary artery and cause sudden death. There is a 50% mortality rate associated with this condition.

Severe chest pain, breathlessness, cyanosis and shock may occur with massive embolism. These problems may be absent with small emboli. An electrocardiogram and lung scan are performed. Relief of pain is important; morphia may be necessary. Oxygen is given at four litres/minute via an MC mask. The treatment of pulmonary embolus is the same as that for deep vein thrombosis.

PROBLEMS ASSOCIATED WITH LOSS OF CONSCIOUSNESS

Predisposing causes

Overdose
– drugs.
– alcohol.
Anaesthetic
Cerebrovascular accident
Cerebral tumours
Head injury
Epilepsy
Liver failure

Infections
– meningitis.
– encephalitis.
– systemic infections.
Hypoglycaemia
Electrolyte imbalance
Respiratory distress
Renal failure (uraemia)
Endocrine disease

Problem 1

Inability to maintain own airway.

Aim

To maintain a clear airway and ensure an adequate oxygen supply to all tissues.

Actions

- Remove dentures.
- Position the person so that the tongue does not fall backwards.
- Place the person in a semi-prone or lateral position.
- Alter the person's position at least two-hourly to prevent stasis in the lungs.
- Perform pharyngeal or tracheal suction to clear secretions.
- Observe the person to detect deterioration in respiratory rate and depth.
- Observe the person to detect the development of cyanosis.

If there is respiratory embarrassment, a Guedal airway can be inserted. Severe respiratory distress may necessitate insertion of an endotracheal tube, the formation of a tracheostomy or mechanical ventilation.

Problem 2

Susceptibility to pressure sores.

Aim

To prevent formation of pressure sores.

Action

See page 39.

Problem 3

Inability to maintain personal hygiene.

Aim

To maintain cleanliness of skin, hair, nails, mouth, and eyes.

Actions

- Wash and dry skin.
- Keep nails clean and short.
- Comb hair regularly and wash as necessary.
- Perform mouth care at least two-hourly.
- Clean eyes with sterile cotton wool balls soaked in warm isotonic saline.
- Prevent risk of injury to eyes due to loss of corneal reflexes (these protect the eyes).
- Shave men daily.

Problem 4

Inability to maintain nutritional state.

Aim

To provide adequate nutrition and fluids.

Action

Feed the person in liquid form via a nasogastric tube or by an intravenous route (See Chapter 9.)

Problem 5

Urinary incontinence or retention.

Aim

To prevent occurrence of incontinence and retention.

Actions

- Express the person's bladder manually every two hours.
- Use appliances:
  - condoms.
  - catheterization.
- Reduce risk of urinary tract infection by strict aseptic catheterization procedure with catheter hygiene at least four-hourly.
- Adequate fluid intake.

Problem 6

Constipation or faecal incontinence.

Aim

To achieve a regular bowel action based on the person's normal habits.

Actions

- Give enemas or suppositories every three days.
- Manually evacuate the bowel.
- Add bran to nasogastric feeds.
- Avoid secondary infection via nasogastric feeds.

Problem 7

Immobility.

Aim

To prevent stiffening of joints, contractures, muscle wasting, foot drop and venous thrombosis. To prevent stasis of secretions, which may lead to chest infection, and of urine, which may lead to urinary calculi formation.

Actions

- Perform passive exercises to all joints each time the person is turned, i.e. at least two-hourly.
- Assist with chest physiotherapy.
- Maintain fluid intake (1500–2000 ml) every 24 hours.

Observation of vital signs will be essential in the unconscious person.

Note the importance of communication. Always speak to the person, call them by their name, tell them what is happening, e.g. when their feeds are being given and when they are being turned. Touch is an important method of communication and should be used as much as possible. Encourage family and friends to come in and talk to the person; they will need continual support. The personal care of the person should be performed with dignity and without unnecessary exposure.

FURTHER READING

CANAVAN, T. (1986). The function of sleep. *Nursing*, **3**, No. 9, 333–334.

CLARK, M. & KADHORN, H. (1988). The nursing prevention of pressure sores in hospital and community patients. *Journal of Advanced Nursing*, **13**, 365–373

HIBBS, P. J. (1989). The economies of pressure sore prevention. *Care of the Critically Ill*, **5**(6), 247–250.

JAHANSHAHS, M. (1986). Insomnia. *Nursing*, **3**, No. 9, 328–332.

JUDD, M. (1989). *Mobility—Patient Problems and Nursing Care*, 1st edn. Heinemann Nursing, Oxford.

LASK, S. (1986). The nurse's role in nutrition education. *Nursing*, **3**, No. 7, 296–300.

LOVE, C. (1990). Deep vein thrombosis—threat to recovery. *Nursing Times*, 86, 31 January, 40–43.

LOVE, C. (1990). Deep vein thrombosis—methods of prevention. *Nursing Times*, 86, 7 February, 52–55.

MILLAZO, V. & RESH, C. (1982). A new approach to the problems of immobilization. *Journal of Neurosurgical Nursing*, **14**(3), 120–123.

PRITCHARD, D. A. & WALKER, V. A. (eds.) (1984). *The Royal Marsden Hospital Manual of Clinical Nursing Policies and Procedures*. Harper and Row, London.

RANKIN BOX, D. F. (1986). Comfort. *Nursing*, Series 3, No. 8, 340–342.

STARLING, M. *et al.* (1990). Project improves practice. (Research project on prevalence and prevention of pressure sores.) *Nursing Times*, 86, 7 February, 40–41.

WATERLOW, J. (1991). A policy that protects. The Waterlow Pressure Sore Prevention/Treatment Policy. *Professional Nurse*, **6**, Issue 5, 258–264.

4   Nursing people with an infection

Infection occurs when a sufficient number of pathogenic (disease-producing) organisms reach a susceptible site, multiply and cause adverse reactions in a person. In order for this process to take place a chain or sequence of events must take place. This chain is made up of a causative agent, a reservoir in which the agent can multiply, a mode of escape from this reservoir, a mode of transmission, a mode of entry and a susceptible host.

The organisms which are capable of producing infection include bacteria, viruses, fungi, protozoa and parasitic worms.

ORGANISMS WHICH PRODUCE INFECTION

Bacteria

These are found in a wide variety of places. They can be present in air, water, soil and food and are also present in some body cavities and on the body surface. They are classified according to their shape: cocci (spherical), bacilli (rod-shaped) or spirochaetes (spiral). They are a major form of disease and can cause serious problems for an individual. Some bacteria are dependent on oxygen (aerobic), while others can live without oxygen (anaerobic). Many bacteria are not pathogenic and some are part of the body's natural defences. These are known as commensals. However, these bacteria may become pathogenic if they gain access to parts of the body that they normally do not inhabit.

Viruses

Viruses are the smallest of the pathogenic organisms and can only be seen under electron-microscopic enlargement. They cause disease by reproducing inside a living cell. The body's normal defence mechanism may destroy the virus, or the virus may spread to other cells, causing problems. In some cases the immediate effects of the invasion of a virus may disappear but the virus remains dormant within the cell and can be reactivated later as the result of a particular stimulus.

Fungi

Fungi are mould-like organisms which produce diseases which are commonly referred to as mycosis. These are usually local infections and it is rare for general infection to occur. Thrush and ringworm are examples of fungal infections.

Protozoa

These are single-celled organisms and are more complex in their structure than bacteria. Malaria, amoebic dysentery and sleeping sickness are examples of protozoal infections.

Parastic worms

Infections may be caused by parasitic worms invading body tissues or organs. These worms are referred to as helminths. Infections caused by helminths tend to occur in tropical areas rather than the United Kingdom. Tapeworm, the filarial worm (flukes) and hookworm are examples of helminths.

NATURAL AND ACQUIRED DEFENCES

The human being has two forms of defence against pathogenic organisms: natural and acquired.

Natural or innate defences

The whole body can be described as a system of defence set up to deter infection. Skin acts as an effective barrier against organisms and the acidic content of its glandular secretions may destroy or inhibit the growth of certain pathogens. Mucous membrane of the respiratory tract helps to trap and carry away organisms. The mucus in the gastrointestinal tract protects the mucous membrane lining from hydrochloric acid and digestive enzymes. Vaginal secretions produce an acidity that causes a resistance to infective agents.

Certain blood cells such as leucocytes and macrophages are designed to engulf and destroy invading pathogens. This is known as phagocytosis. Lymph nodes are situated along the course of the lymphatic system to filter out the bacteria destroyed by phagocytosis. Blood and body fluids contain enzymes, known as lysozymes, that destroy bacteria, and gammaglobulins which form antibodies in response to infective agents or their toxins.

These are just some examples of the way that the whole body can be regarded as a natural defence system. Unfortunately, in ill-health, or through surgical intervention, or the use of tubes and cannulae, we in hospital breach these defences, making it more likely that infection will occur.

Natural immunity to certain pathogens also varies with species, race and individuals.

Acquired defences

Immunity to an infection can occur as the result of the individual coming into contact with an infecting agent. A person may develop immunity by forming antibodies or sensitized T-lymphocytes. This can take place naturally, as for example when antibodies developed by the mother are passed through the placenta to a fetus, or can be artificially induced. Artificial passive immunity is conferred by injecting serum, taken from another organism, which has actively developed immune bodies to a particular infection. This form of immunity may only last for a period of time and so will need to be repeated. Tetanus antitoxin and human immune globulin are examples of this form of immunity.

If a person's immunity to infection breaks down, then infection with its resulting problems occurs. Acquired immune deficiency syndrome (AIDS) is an example of this. It is caused by the human immunodeficiency virus (HIV) which attacks and may destroy T4 lymphocytes. Without this form of lymphocyte, cells are particularly susceptible to infections and rare forms of carcinoma such as Kaposi's sarcoma.

FACTORS THAT PREDISPOSE A PERSON TO AN INFECTION

- Age. Infants, children and older people are more susceptible to infection.
- Nutrition. Malnourishment means that people are more likely to develop infections. This is particularly true if their diet has been deficient in proteins and vitamins, as these are necessary for the body to develop its natural antibodies.
- Exposure to cold. A lowered body temperature causes physiological changes such as reduction in blood supply to the tissues and a suppression of antibody formation, which mean that the person's natural immunity is lowered.

- Occupation. Certain occupations may mean an increased exposure to infective agents or may lower the body's natural immunity. People who work in coal mines are an example.
- Ill-health. Diseases can weaken the body's natural immunity, and so make infection more likely. A person who has diabetes mellitus is more likely, if they have hyperglycaemia, to develop infection. So too can the blood cancers of white blood cells—leukaemia.
- Admission to hospital, radiation and drug therapy. Admission to hospital is potentially hazardous from the perspective of infection (see page 19). As a result of ill-health, people may undergo radiation therapy. This can suppress bone marrow, leucocyte and antibody production and so make a person more likely to develop infection. Certain drugs, notably corticosteroids and immunosuppressive drugs, may suppress the production of lymphocytes and antibodies. A person is therefore at more risk of developing infection.

NURSING PEOPLE WITH AN INFECTION IN HOSPITAL

A hospital environment presents a high risk for infection. In earlier times death from infection was so high that it led to a surgeon, John Bell, in the early 1800s, to write to his fellow surgeons: 'Let us bear in mind that this is a hospital disease; that without the circle of the infected walls men are safe; let us therefore hurry them out of this house of death . . . let us lay them in a school room, a church, on a dunghill or in a stable . . . let us carry them anywhere but to their graves'. This high mortality rate from infection was at the basis of Florence Nightingales's famous saying: 'The first requirement of a hospital is that it should do the sick no harm.'

Hospitals remain sources of infection. We put people together in close proximity, some of whom have infections and some of whom have lowered resistance to infection due to ill-health. We then breach or lower their natural defences against infection. This can be through surgery, the insertion of catheters, intravenous cannulae and other equipment. They may also require drugs and radiation which add to a lowered natural resistance. We often move them around this setting—to X-ray departments, operating theatres and investigative units.

Within this system they are then cared for by a large number and variety of different people. They will come into contact with people such as nurses, physiotherapists, phlebotomists, medical staff and occupational therapists. Many of these people will be touching them and carrying out procedures where infection may be introduced. We may have to carry out our care in unsuitable environments. The numbers of lavatories and wash basins, the construction of the sluice and access to a treatment room, may be inadequate.

To add to the risk, a series of relatives and friends will then visit the ward environment. They may have come from work or shopping and may have a mild infection themselves.

Perhaps it is, then, not surprising that hospital-acquired infection can take place. Some studies suggest that 10% of all people admitted to hospital acquire an infection that they did not have on arrival. The commonest acquired infections are urinary tract infections, chest infections and wound infections. There are now also infections which are acquired which are resistant to many antibiotics. Some of these infections are in danger of becoming endemic within hospitals. One of these, which remains a source of concern, is infection caused by multi-resistant *Staphylococcus aureus*.

THE ROLE OF THE NURSE IN LESSENING THE RISK OF CROSS-INFECTION

Education and teaching of other nurses, other health professionals, relatives and the person admitted to hospital

The nurse has an important role in teaching about cross-infection, procedures involving asepsis, wound management, sources of infection and nursing procedures where cross-infection is a risk. These include urinary catheter care, the collection of specimens, changing of infusions and assistance with hygiene. Patients and relatives will need advice on areas such as not touching wounds, managing urinary catheters correctly, hygiene and the risk of visiting if a relative or friend has an infection.

In addition, other health professionals may need education about cross-infection, particularly in respect of touching dressings, looking at wounds and general hygiene.

Provision of a safe ward environment

The nurse has an important role in ensuring that the ward environment is conducive to reducing the risk of cross-infection. Areas that need consideration are the organization of the sluice, the provision of suitable containers for the removal of infected matter, sufficient handwashing facilities, the supply of sterile equipment and adequate facilities for isolation nursing.

Teamwork

Nurses must liaise with medical staff about any changes in a person's condition that indicate infection may be developing. They should also discuss with microbiologists the results of any specimens and swabs that are required. In addition, if the hospital has a clinical nurse specialist in infection control, then their involvement with ward nursing staff is critical.

Communication

Nursing instructions about the management of procedures where potential infection is present should be clear and concise. Nursing care plans should state what sort of dressing should be performed. It is also important that the progress notes contain a comment on the nature of the wound and its healing. Similarly, care plans should state when a person is at risk of infection and the actions that the nurse should carry out to detect the development of infection.

Organization of nursing within a ward environment

Nurses have a role in ensuring that nursing is organized in a way that lessens the risk of cross-infection. Areas that should be considered are: when bed-making should take place, where and when wound dressings should be performed and how hygiene bowls should be stored. Dressings to wounds should not be performed during periods when beds are being made, due to the increased organisms in the air during this procedure. Where possible, wound dressings should be carried out in a treatment room. Hygiene bowls should be stored upside down on a person's locker and the same bowl used for the duration of that person's stay in hospital.

Role model

The nurse should ensure that their own hygiene is good and that their uniform is clean. Their own practice of asepsis should be correct, as it serves as a powerful method of education for junior nurses. A nurse should also ensure that their own knowledge of cross-infection and nursing procedures involving asepsis is up to date and based on nursing research. They should also be knowledgeable about their own hospital's isolation procedures.

Nurses have an important responsibility in any situation where infection exists, or there is a risk of infection developing, to promote and practise measures that prevent cross-infection to those they are caring for, their relatives, nursing colleagues and other members of the hospital staff.

CONTROL OF CROSS-INFECTION BY ISOLATION

Some people who develop an infection are at particular risk of infecting others and so isolation nursing may be required. There are three categories of isolation: standard isolation, excretion/secretion isolation and strict isolation. In addition, there is a group of people at particular risk of developing an infection and who may require isolation nursing to protect them from other people. This is known as protective isolation.

Standard isolation is used for infecting agents where the route of transmission is direct contact, air or dust.

Excretion/secretion isolation is used where infection may be spread by a person's faeces, urine, blood or amniotic fluid.

Strict isolation is used for highly transmissible dangerous infections which, although rare, may easily be spread to other people. General hospitals do not have facilities for this form of isolation and people need to be transferred to a specialist isolation hospital.

Protective isolation is used for people who, either because of their disease or the treatment they are having, are highly susceptible to infection. This can be caused by their own normal bacteria (auto-infection), or be derived from staff, other patients, relatives and friends, or the inanimate ward environment.

Hospitals have now developed guidelines for each of these categories of isolation. These policies should consider the following areas within each type of isolation:

- Preparation of the room. What equipment is necessary in a room for the type of isolation to be used?
- Protective clothing. Instructions on whether aprons or gowns, masks and gloves are required should be stated.
- Hand hygiene. When hands should be washed and with what solution should be stated.
- Disposal of potentially infected items. Instructions should be clear as to how dressings, refuse, urine, faeces, bed linen, needles, disposable syringes, sterile equipment and crockery and cutlery should be disposed.
- Laboratory specimens. The policy should state how specimens that are required should be sent to the laboratory and whether they require a 'high-risk' label to be attached.
- Transporting patients. If people need to attend other departments or areas of the hospital the policy should make it clear how this can be safely carried out.
- Visitors. The policy should state what instructions visitors should follow if they wish to visit a person on isolation. It should also state whether visiting inside a room is permitted.
- Decontamination after a person has gone home. The policy for each type of isolation should state how the room and the equipment within it is to be cleaned when a person no longer requires isolation.
- Death. The procedure to be followed in the event of a person dying while in isolation should also be stated.

The particular problems a person will have and the nursing care that they will require will depend on the reasons for their isolation and their individual health/ill-health. However, people in isolation, and their families, may suffer from feelings associated with this form of nursing.

The nurse should remember that it is the organism that is being isolated and not the person. We need to assess the person for their perception of the reason for isolation and the feelings that it engenders. Isolation can be frightening and feelings of rejection and depression may occur. Time should be taken to explore these feelings and plan nursing actions to relieve any actual or potential problems. This should include the family, who may be experiencing their own fears and anxieties.

It is of particular importance that nursing does not centre on physical care. We may only feel that we should go in the side room because a person requires a particular aspect of physical care. It is of equal importance that we spend time with a person, listening, sharing thoughts and discussing their feelings. We, perhaps, may ourselves be worried that we may develop the infection that the person is suffering from. Understanding the type of infection and, in particular, its mode of transmission, can help alleviate these fears.

People on protective isolation also have their own series of fears and anxieties. They may have leukaemia and be on a powerful cytoxic regime of drug therapy. Or they may have had a transplant of an organ and, due to the drugs used to prevent the rejection of the transplanted organ, be particularly susceptible to infection. Fears about death, or what happens if the organ transplant does not work, may be present. In addition, relatives may not be permitted in the room and may only be allowed to communicate using a telephone outside the room. The nurse must assess the feelings that are occurring and plan the care that is required for that individual.

NOTIFIABLE DISEASES

Some infections are classified as notifiable diseases. This means that the appropriate medical officer of the local environmental health department must be informed. This is required under the Public Health (Control of Disease) Act 1984. The list of diseases to be notified is modified as new infectious diseases arise. Infectious diseases which must be notified are:

Acute encephalitis	Measles
Acute meningitis	Mumps
Acute poliomyelitis	Ophthalmia neonatorum
Anthrax	Paratyphoid fever
Cholera	Rabies
Diphtheria	Relapsing fever
Dysentery	Rubella
Food poisoning (all sources)	Scarlet fever
	Smallpox
Infective jaundice	Tetanus
Lassa fever	Tuberculosis
Leprosy	Typhoid fever
Leptospirosis	Viral haemorrhagic fevers
Malaria	Whooping cough
Marburg disease	Yellow fever

Although not required by Statute, it is recommended that *Campylobacter* gastroenteritis, meningococcal septicaemia and Legionnaire's disease are also notified to the appropriate community medical officer.

Certain sexually transmitted diseases must also be

reported so that contacts can be traced. This mechanism is different to that of notifiable diseases.

Although there has been a decline in the incidence of communicable diseases within the United Kingdom due to health education and immunization, they do remain endemic in parts of the world.

Detailed information on particular infectious diseases, their method of spread, incubation period, infectious period, problems, complications and forms of intervention are available in more specialist textbooks (see Further reading).

CONCLUSION

Nurses have an important role to play within community and hospital settings in relation to health education. As the incidence of certain infectious diseases lessens, complacency can set in and the importance of immunization may become diminished. There is concern that the number of children being immunized in the United Kingdom is falling. Health visitors, school nurses and other community nurses have an important role in education as to the importance of immunization and the problems that infectious diseases can cause.

In addition, the incidence of sexually transmitted diseases continues to increase. Non-specific urethritis and HIV are both increasing. Health education in this area is of vital importance.

Hospital-acquired infection remains a problem. It causes unnecessary suffering which may be physical and psychological and have economic and social consequences for the individual. It also has economic consequences for the Health Service, with the increased length of time a person stays in hospital and the extra resources that are required to treat the acquired infection. Nurses have an important role in preventing cross-infection within hospital and to ensure that Florence Nightingale's statement, that the 'Hospital should do the patient no harm', continues to guide our professional knowledge and practice.

FURTHER READING

AYLIFFE, G. A. J., GEDDES, A. M. & WILLIAMS, J. D. (1981). *Control of Hospital Infection*, 2nd edn. Chapman and Hall, London.
BENN, R. A. V. (1986). *Aids to Microbiology and Infectious Diseases*. Churchill Livingstone, Edinburgh and London.
Immunisation against Hepatitis B. (1987). Report of the Board of Science and Education, British Medical Association, 1st edn. Chameleon Press, London.
Introducing Immunology. Open Learning for Nurses (1987). (Behavioural Science Series), 1st edn. H. Charlesworth and Co., Huddersfield.
JOINT COMMITTEE ON VACCINATION AND IMMUNISATION. *Immunisation against Infectious Diseases*. Department of Health and Social Security, Welsh Office, Scottish Home and Health Department.
KIRKIS E. J. & GRIER, M. A. (1988). *Nurses Guide to Infection Control Practice*. W.B. Saunders, London.
PALMER, M. B. (1984). *Infection Control*. Saunders Blue Book Series. W.B. Saunders, London.
PARKER, J. & STUCKE, U. (1982). *Microbiology for Nurses*, 6th edn. Baillière Tindall, London.
PARRY, W. H. (1979). *Communicable Diseases*, 3rd edn. Hodder and Stoughton, London.

5   Caring for the dying person and their family

The period of dying may be accompanied by pain, bodily impairment and mental anguish. It is difficult for a person to visualize their own death, and most people have a greater fear of the *process of dying* than the *fact of death*. The nurse has an important role in allaying these fears and anxieties.

Where possible it is best for people who are dying to be cared for at home. Familiar surroundings and the nearness of those who are aware of the individual's needs and preferences can ease the fear felt. Support can be given by the community nurses or the domiciliary nurses attached to hospices.

Recent years have seen the development of hospices for the terminally ill. These are centres specializing in the care of people who are dying. They provide a model on which nurses within hospitals should base their care.

There is perhaps a danger that, instead of learning from these specialist centres, nurses will leave the proper care of the dying to them, the thinking being that if you have a renal disease you go to a renal unit, and if you are dying you go to a hospice. However, as most deaths take place within a hospital setting, nurses must not abandon their role in these circumstances. Caring for people who are dying is an integral part of nursing. The skills and attitudes developed in the hospice movement can be used to give good care within hospital wards.

The aim of this chapter is to outline some of the ways in which a nurse can help the person who is dying. The areas that will be considered are:

- Psychological care
- Spiritual care
- Family involvement and support
- 'To tell or not to tell'
- The needs of the nursing staff
- Physical care

PSYCHOLOGICAL CARE

The psychological response to dying involves certain characteristic stages. Dr Elizabeth Kübler-Ross has described five stages of grief a person may experience on learning they have fatal illness. They are defence mechanisms, and an awareness of these stages will help the nurse to anticipate and alleviate the person's fears.

Denial

People develop the feeling that 'it can't be true'. This enables them to collect themselves and come to terms with the information. Denial is normally a holding pattern and will soon be replaced by partial acceptance.

Nursing intervention

Listening is important at this stage. People should be allowed to day-dream about happier things. Denial will fade if they are aware that someone will be available to help them express their feelings when they are ready.

Anger

When denial fades it can be replaced by anger and rage— 'Why me?' This anger may be directed at many different things. Nurses are often the target for this anger and 'can do nothing right'. It is almost as if the person is saying 'I'm not dead yet'.

Nursing intervention

This is a difficult period as the anger will be directed towards all sorts of things: the food may be poor, the bed badly made, the nurses may do everything wrong, the doctors don't know what they are talking about, and so on. The nurse must remember why the person is angry. The anger must not be taken personally. It is a generalized feeling of frustration and rage which is displaced onto individual things and people.

It is important to understand what is happening and to give the person time to express emotion. Anger will then fade. It is all too easy to take this behaviour personally, and to avoid the person, but this may only increase anger as it leaves no one to attack. The provision of time and attention will allow the person to work through their feelings.

Bargaining

This is a stage where people may try to enter into an agreement with someone or something in an attempt to postpone the inevitable. It is usually a brief period.

Nursing intervention

Many of the bargains may be unexpressed. Individuals may make them with themselves, or with their God. The nurse must ensure that spiritual needs are being met, and this may be an appropriate time to involve the relevant religious authority or adviser.

Depression

Denial and anger may be replaced by a great sense of loss or sadness. This is perhaps a preparatory grief that the person needs to suffer before final separation. It may focus on a past or impending loss.

Nursing intervention

The nurse must allow time for grieving. Non-verbal communication can be particularly helpful. Sitting with people and holding their hands can mean more than words; so can the expression on one's face. Again, providing time is important. Encouragement, assurance and telling people not to feel sad is *unhelpful*. They will naturally be sad and one should share that feeling and not deny its validity. These feelings are necessary if the person is to reach the final stage of acceptance.

Acceptance

A person who has had the time and help to work through these stages will reach a point when they are neither depressed nor angry. Having expressed rage and a sense of loss, they reach a stage of quiet acceptance. This is not a stage of giving up, but a period almost void of feelings.

Nursing intervention

This stage is often characterized by tiredness, weakness and long periods of sleep. Again, non-verbal communication is vital. Sitting in silence with the person to show them that you are still there and that you care is important. Touching, holding hands or straightening pillows will help provide comfort.

These stages do not always occur in sequence and may overlap each other. An awareness of these defence mechanisms should guide the nurse's approach and care.

Throughout these stages it is important that the nurse allows the person the time and the opportunity to express feelings. It is all too easy for nursing to be reduced to the completion of physical tasks, while the nurse, with their own anxieties, avoids the psychological care of the individual.

If possible, nursing people in side rooms should be avoided. This arrangement can make it too easy for nurses to go in, complete their tasks and leave, avoiding the person. People are often nursed in side rooms to allay the anxieties of the nursing staff, rather than for their own benefit. Care and involvement should be *increased* and not withdrawn because someone is terminally ill.

SPIRITUAL CARE

People's spiritual needs may be of the greatest importance to them during this period. A nurse should know from the nursing assessment and from their relationship with the person, whether they have religious beliefs.

In our multi-cultural society, religious beliefs vary considerably. If a nurse is unable to meet and help with any individual's beliefs, it is important that they ensure they are met by others. Members of the family may be able to provide spiritual support. More particularly, the relevant religious authority or adviser should be involved. In addition to helping the person and their family directly, they will provide guidance for the nurses so as to ensure that their nursing intervention conforms to the person's religious beliefs.

FAMILY INVOLVEMENT AND SUPPORT

The nurse cannot give valid help and support to the person who is dying unless they also consider the family. Their feelings will include hopelessness, anger, isolation and sadness. They may well experience some or all of the psychological stages mentioned previously. Unless the family's feelings are expressed and understood, the individual will be nursed in a vacuum. The care of them as a whole person will suffer accordingly.

Psychological support can be given by involving the family in physical care. Carrying out certain procedures and tasks can ease feelings of helplessness. Washing, positioning, giving medication and making beds, for example, can be done by a nurse and a member of the family together. They should be directly involved in caring. It must always be remembered that the dying person is their spouse, child or other close relative.

The spouse is often the first person to be informed of the severity of the illness and to be told that death may occur. He or she is often then left, without support, to tell the rest of the family. The nurse can help by informing and involving all the family.

The nurse must provide the time to listen to family anxieties and emotions, and must be able to explain what is happening. They should also act as a bridge between the person who is dying and their family, helping them to communicate with each other. The person who is dying may be able to help the family accept their situation by discussing feelings with them.

Difficulties with visiting, staying at the hospital, leaving children at home, finances or legal concerns can all cause anxiety at such a time. The involvement of social workers or other members of the family may help to ease these worries.

The nurse should also be aware of what support there will be for the immediate family after the death. Bereavement counselling and support from social workers can help ease the feelings that will occur. The nurse must remember that the family's feelings will not end with the person's death.

The degree of family involvement and support will obviously vary on each occasion. The principle remains, however, that, without their involvement, the care of the patient will suffer.

'TO TELL OR NOT TO TELL'

Should people who are dying be told? This is a question often raised in nursing. Kübler-Ross says that the question should not be 'Should we tell them what is wrong?', but rather, 'How can we share this information with the person?' This approach is admirable. It establishes a different relationship to that which commonly exists. One can listen to the person for cues about their willingness to know more. It is an empathetic way of relating, developing a relationship based on confidence and trust.

It is important that this sharing of knowledge is accompanied by an assurance that the person will not be abandoned. They must be reassured that everything possible will still be done to maintain their dignity and relieve specific problems.

Both Elizabeth Kübler-Ross and Cicely Saunders (see Further reading list) would argue that the majority of people are aware of their impending death, whether they have been told or not. People pick up this knowledge from the behaviour of their family, the nurses and the doctors. They can sense a change in approach and any tendency to avoid them and their problems.

Given these facts, the nurse should constantly be aware

of how much information the person wishes to share, and should always be sensitive to the timing of communication. The concept of sharing knowledge means that some people will know explicitly and others implicitly what is wrong. This is not telling lies but sharing knowledge according to the wishes of the person who is dying.

THE NEEDS OF THE NURSING STAFF

Caring for the dying creates anxiety and stress among nurses. They may have had little or no experience of death; their own feelings may be unexplored and their means of supporting one another are often poor. As a result, the care they provide for those who are dying may be inadequate.

Within the setting of a ward, nursing staff can share feelings in a supportive way. Discussing what one feels— be it anger, impotence, helplessness, sadness, or a combination of any of these—is necessary when caring for a person who is dying. This must be done openly. Many feelings can be difficult to express as people are worried about what others will think—'How can I say I dislike or get fed up with someone who is dying?' These feelings may be experienced by others, and only by discussing them together and sharing them can nurses give each other help and support. This can be done either on a one-to-one basis or at meetings of ward staff.

Nurses must be aware of the stress they will experience when nursing people who are dying, and of the emotional demands with which they will have to cope. Unless nurses can discuss and explore their feelings, the care they give will suffer.

PHYSICAL CARE

The person who is dying may have a variety of physical

problems caused by their disease (or diseases). Common problems include:

pain	lethargy and weakness
anorexia	pressure sores
nausea and vomiting	insomnia
dry mouth	constipation
hiccough	diarrhoea
dyspnoea	urinary frequency
cough	urinary incontinence

The nursing intervention for these problems is outlined in Chapter 3.

The role of the nurse is vital in the context of these problems, and involves constant assessment and observation. The dying person's general condition means that specific problems can arise very suddenly. The nurse must continually assess the person to anticipate problems. Any problems that cannot be anticipated must be alleviated quickly. This is important, not only to relieve the particular discomfort, but to assure the person that they have not been abandoned. It emphasizes the philosophy that, although nothing can be done to change the final outcome, this does not mean that there is nothing to be done at all.

If nursing and medical intervention can minimize a person's physical suffering, they will then be free to concentrate on other matters.

Pain in people who are dying

Pain in those who are terminally ill serves no useful purpose. The aim of care should be to ensure that no pain is experienced.

Pain is a wholly subjective symptom. It is impossible to devise a system whereby the nurse can determine the degree of pain felt, yet it is necessary to assess the pain in order to ensure it is controlled. The only reliable method is to ask the person.

A pain observation chart has been designed to help make the assessment of pain more systematic. The person is asked about their pain at regular intervals, and the nurse records the location and severity of the pain on the chart. This enables the effectiveness of analgesia to be closely monitored. If analgesia is being given regularly, it is necessary to make an observation with each dose, and another half-way between each dose. This is because analgesia must be organized so as to stop pain being experienced before the next dose is given. The memory or fear of pain returning must be prevented as well as the pain itself.

To use the chart, ask the person to mark *all* their pains on the body diagram (Figure 5.1). It is important to note that pain is often felt in more than one area. Label each site of pain with a letter (A, B, C, etc.). Once this initial assessment has been made, systematic recordings can be carried out on subsequent occasions. At each observation time:

1. Ask the person to assess the pain at each separate site since the last observation. Using the scale with the body diagram (Figure 5.1) enter the number or letter in the appropriate column of the pain chart (Figure 5.2).
2. Record the overall pain since the last observation. Use the same scale and enter the level of pain in the column marked 'overall'.
3. Record what nursing measures have been taken to relieve pain.
4. Record the analgesia given.
5. Note any comment on pain from the person or the nursing staff.

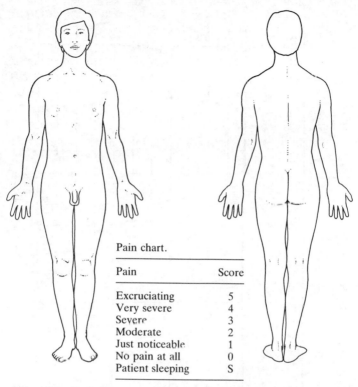

Pain chart.

Pain	Score
Excruciating	5
Very severe	4
Severe	3
Moderate	2
Just noticeable	1
No pain at all	0
Patient sleeping	S

Figure 5.1 Body diagram and scoring system for assessing pain.

This is a means of communication to be used with the person and not on them. It may be helpful if they fill in the chart themselves.

Many terminally ill people suffer from cancer and may experience very severe pain. As a result they may be prescribed powerful analgesics such as diamorphine and morphine.

Analgesia is given orally where possible. If vomiting,

PAIN OBSERVATION CHART

PATIENT
IDENTIFICATION
LABEL

DATE ....

SHEET NUMBER .....

TIME	PAIN RATING									MEASURES TO RELIEVE PAIN									COMMENTS FROM PATIENTS AND/OR STAFF	Initials
	BY SITES								OVER-ALL	ANALGESIC GIVEN (Name, dose, route, time)	Lifting	Turning	Massage	Distracting activities*	Position change*	Additional aids*	Other*			
	A	B	C	D	E	F	G	H												

Specify where starred

Figure 5.2 Pain chart.

weakness or dysphagia makes this difficult, drugs can be given rectally or by injection. Where injections are required, they no longer need to be given every three or four hours, but can be given by a syringe pump. A 24-hour dose of an analgesic drug is drawn into a syringe, to which a cannula with a butterfly needle is attached. This syringe is fitted into a pump, which is set to compress the syringe barrel at a steady rate and empty the syringe over 24 hours. The butterfly needle is inserted subcutaneously, and the pump may be fitted into a holster or pouch which fits under the arm or around the waist (Figure 5.3). Excellent pain control can be achieved by this method. The analgesic usually used is diamorphine. The syringe is recharged each day and the needle site is altered after 48 hours.

In addition to the wide choice of analgesic drugs available, the nurse must not neglect the range of nursing measures which help to alleviate pain (see page 43).

The importance of pain control cannot be overstated. Pain can be the most important problem for the person who is dying, clouding everything else.

CONCLUSION

Wherever possible, people should be nursed at home and cared for by their families. The environment is familiar and the person is appreciated as an individual. Anxieties and fears will be reduced. However, only a small number of dying people can be cared for in this way. Most deaths take place within a hospital, and therefore nurses have a responsibility to become skilled at caring for people who are dying.

It must *never* be assumed that terminal care consists merely of routines performed when there is nothing more

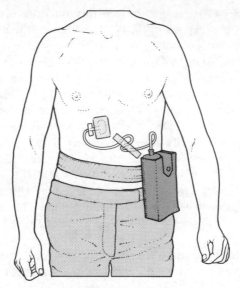

Figure 5.3 Continuous analgesia.

to be done. It should not be seen as the end-product of
failed medical treatment. If this is allowed to happen, the
person will feel abandoned and their deepest needs will be
ignored. Rather, nurses should try to provide positive
help during this period of life.

Caring for people who will recover alongside those
who will not is sometimes regarded as impossible. Care,
however, is individual. Nurses must learn to adapt their
care to the needs of each person and avoid employing a
generalized, blanket approach. In order to do this they
must understand the specific physical and psychological
needs of the individual who is dying. This understanding
must involve the members of the family, each of whom
will also have their own particular needs.

Nurses have a positive role in allaying anxiety and fears

about the process of dying. They have the opportunity to help the person live this part of their life without physical distress and with dignity.

This can only be an introduction to caring for people and their families who are dying. All nurses should continue to develop their knowledge, skills and attitudes through further reading, their educational programme and experience. In particular, they should learn from nurses skilled in this aspect of nursing. Within both hospital and community settings there are now Macmillan nurses who nurse as specialists within this area. In addition to providing skilled, sensitive support for people and their families, they are excellent role models for other nurses By using them for advice and guidance we can develop our own skills and expertise in this area of nursing and so provide better care for people and their families through this period of their lives.

FURTHER READING

CASTLES, M. R. & MURRAY, R. B. (1979). *Dying in an Institution: Nurse Patient Perspectives*. Appleton-Century Crofts, New York.

COOK & OLTJENBRUNS. (1989). *Dying and Grieving, Lifespan and Family Perspective*. Holt, Rinehart and Winston, New York.

ERIKSSON, J. H. (1989). *Oncology Nursing* (Springhouse Notes), Springhouse Publishing Co., Springhouse Pennsylvania.

HECTOR, W. & WHITFIELD, S. (1982). *Nursing Care for the Dying Patient and the Family*. William Heineman Medical Books, London.

KUBLER-ROSS, E. (1973). *On Death and Dying*. Tavistock, London.

LAMERTON, R. (1980). *Care of the Dying*. Richard Clay (The Chaucer Press Ltd), Bungay, Suffolk.

MCGILLOWAY, O. & MYCO, F. (1985). *Nursing and Spiritual Care*. Lippincot Nursing Services. Harper and Row, London.

NEUBERGER, J. (1987). *Caring for Dying People of Different Faiths*. Austin Cornish Lisa Saintsbury Foundation, London.

Nursing Skill Books (1987). *Dealing with Death and Dying*, 2nd edn. Spring House Publishing Co., Springhouse Pennsylvania.

PARKS, C. M. (1987). *Bereavement Studies of Grief in Adult Life*. Penguin Books, Harmondsworth.

ROBBINS, J. (ed.) (1983). *Caring for the Dying Patient and their Family*. Harper and Row, London.

SAUNDERS, C. (1978). *The Management of Terminal Disease*. Edward Arnold, London.

SAUNDERS, C., SUMMERS, D. H. & TELLER, N. (1983). *Hospice, the Living Idea*. Edward Arnold, London.

STEDEFORTH, A. (1984). *Facing Death, Patients' Families and Professionals*. William Heineman Medical Books, London.

6   Nursing people with problems of their cardiovascular system

The cardiovascular system consists of the heart and blood vessels. Figure 6.1 shows the chambers of the heart and the great vessels that enter and leave the heart.

There are three layers of the heart:

pericardium—outer sac of two coats
myocardium—muscle tissue
endocardium—lining

The coronary arteries, which supply the myocardium with blood, are shown in Figure 6.2.

Contraction of the atria and ventricles is caused by electrical impulses passing along the conducting pathways of the heart.

INVESTIGATIONS

Electrocardiogram

An electrocardiogram (ECG) is the tracing obtained by recording the electrical impulses conducted in the heart muscle. Figure 6.3 shows a normal ECG.

Echocardiogram

An echocardiogram is a recording of sound waves reflected from surfaces outside and inside the heart. Valve

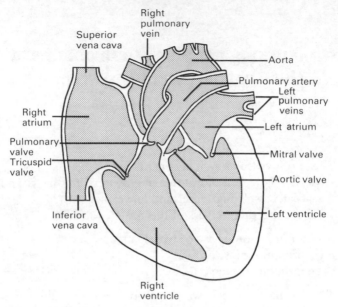

Figure 6.1 The heart.

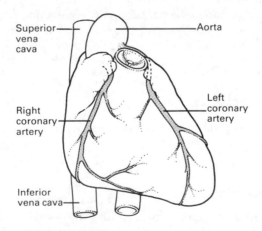

Figure 6.2 The coronary arteries.

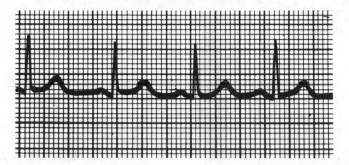

Figure 6.3 Normal ECG.

disease can be diagnosed using this technique. The size of the ventricles can also be assessed.

Cardiac catheterization

This procedure involves the passage of a thin, hollow, flexible tube (catheter) into the right or left side of the heart. The catheter is inserted into a vein or artery of the arm or leg. The catheter is radio-opaque and so its insertion can be monitored using X-rays. This technique is used in order to measure the pressures in the vessels and chambers of the heart. Blood samples can be taken for blood gas estimations.

A radio-opaque dye can be injected via the catheter to outline the vessels. This procedure is called angiography.

There are risks associated with cardiac catheterization and careful explanation and consent are necessary. A mild sedative is sometimes given prior to the procedure, which is performed under a local anaesthetic. The person should have nothing to eat or drink for six hours before the investigation.

The risks of cardiac catheterization are:

haemorrhage from the site

arrhythmias
infection

The insertion site should be observed every 15 minutes for
the first few hours. The person should stay in bed. Direct
pressure should be applied if bleeding occurs. The pulse
and blood pressure should be recorded every 15 minutes
for two hours and then every 30 minutes for four hours.
Irregularity of the pulse may indicate arrhythmias. The

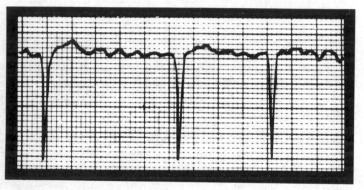

Figure 6.4   Atrial fibrillation.

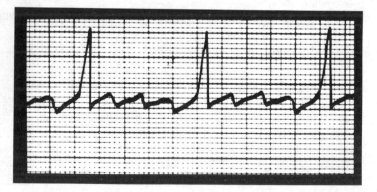

Figure 6.5   Atrial flutter.

doctor should be informed of this and of any episodes of chest pain. The temperature should be recorded every four hours. Pyrexia may indicate infection.

ARRHYTHMIAS

The normal heart beat is regular. Disturbances in heart rhythm are called arrhythmias. Some of the common arrhythmias are shown in Figures 6.4 to 6.8.

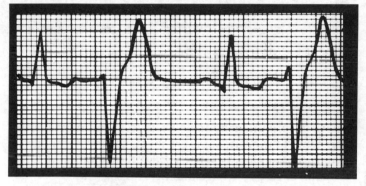

Figure 6.6 Ventricular ectopics.

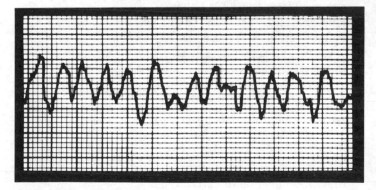

Figure 6.7 Ventricular fibrillation.

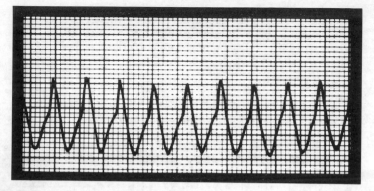

Figure 6.8   Ventricular tachycardia.

CONGENITAL HEART DISEASE

Various forms of abnormality can occur during the development of the heart. Some are mild and can go unnoticed. Some are so severe that the child dies soon after birth. The main types of congenital heart disease are:

Patent ductus arteriosus (Figure 6.9)
Pulmonary valve stenosis (Figure 6.10)
Fallot's tetralogy (Figure 6.11)
– ventricular septal defect
– dextro position of aorta
– pulmonary valve stenosis
– thickened wall of right ventricle
Atrial septal defect (Figure 6.12)

Causes

Maternal infection in early pregnancy,
e.g. rubella or genetic.

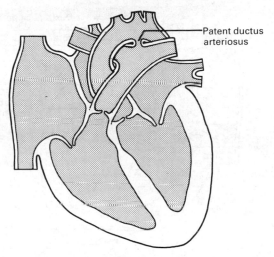

Figure 6.9 Patent ductus arteriosus.

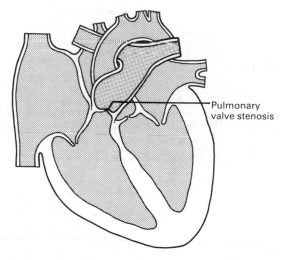

Figure 6.10 Pulmonary valve stenosis.

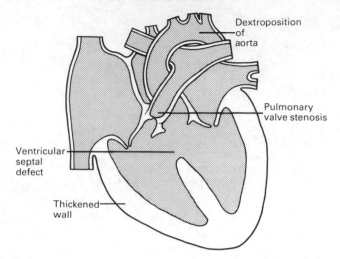

Figure 6.11 Fallot's tetralogy.

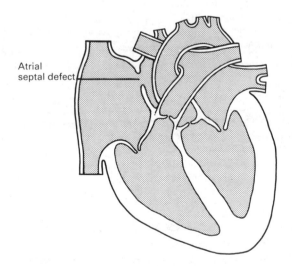

Figure 6.12 Atrial septal defect.

Assessment

- Cyanosis
  - if blood is shunted from right to left side of the heart
- Dyspnoea
- Clubbing of fingers
- Failure to thrive
- Heart murmurs often noticed during a medical examination. Most congenital abnormalities are surgically corrected.

CHRONIC VALVULAR DISEASE

This condition occurs mainly as a result of inflammation of the valve cusps leading to distortion, fibrosis, and calcification of the valve.

Chronic valvular disease often occurs as a result of rheumatic fever (see page 377).

- Stenosis is narrowing of a valve.
- Incompetence is inadequate closure of the valve.
- Regurgitation is backflow of blood as a result of incompetence. Incompetence and regurgitation are often used interchangeably in relation to valvular disease.

Mitral valve disease

There is a history of rheumatic fever in about half the people who develop mitral valve disease. Mitral stenosis is more common than mitral incompetence, although they may occur together.

Congestion of the lungs causes shortness of breath and tiredness, and acute pulmonary oedema may occur. Atrial fibrillation is usually present and right heart failure gradually appears.

Aortic valve disease

Aortic valve disease may be due to congenital malformation, endocarditis, syphilis, or rheumatic heart disease.
Stenosis or incompetence may occur. Both aortic stenosis
and incompetence result in enlargement (hypertrophy) of
the muscle of the left ventricle. Left ventricular failure
eventually occurs, followed by right heart failure.

The main problems are:

– Breathlessness
– Tiredness
– Angina

Pulmonary and tricuspid valve disease

Tricuspid valve disease is usually due to rheumatic heart
disease and is associated with mitral and aortic valve
disease. Pulmonary valve congestion is uncommon and is
usually due to congenital malformation.

Right heart failure results from these conditions. Back
pressure is transmitted via the vena cava into the system
circulation.

Approach to people with valvular disease

For treatment of cardiac failure, see page 118.
Cardiac surgery may be performed and involves either
valvotomy (dilation of the valve) or valve replacements.

The types of valve in use are:

homografts—human tissue
heterografts—non-human tissue, e.g. pig valves
mechanical valves

Anticoagulant therapy is necessary following insertion of
mechanical valves in order to prevent thrombus formation. There is an infection risk associated with this type of
surgery.

People who are preparing to have cardiac surgery require careful explanation about the procedure and their postoperative care. It is helpful if they are able to meet a nurse from the intensive care unit who can provide explanations and be a familiar face postoperatively.

ISCHAEMIC HEART DISEASE

Ischaemic heart disease is caused by a reduction in the blood supply to the heart and is usually due to athero-sclerosis of the coronary arteries. Fatty substances such as cholesterol are deposited in the walls of the arteries, gradually narrowing the lumen. This results in a reduction of the blood supply to the myocardium and the pain known as angina occurs.

A clot of blood (thrombus) may form on the athero-matous plaque and block the artery, drastically reducing the blood supply to the mycocardium. Necrosis of the area of muscle served by the affected artery occurs. This is termed a myocardial infarction.

Coronary heart disease is a leading cause of death in males aged 35 to 65 years; the incidence in women is also increasing. It is a disease of Western countries. A number of risk factors have been implicated:

higher levels of serum cholesterol and triglycerides
smoking
decreased physical activity
stress
hypertension
diabetes

Angina pectoris

Angina is the pain resulting from inadequate blood supply to the myocardium.

Predisposing causes

atherosclerosis
severe anaemia
hypertension
aortic stenosis

In the above conditions the requirements of the myocardium are increassed.

Assessment

Central chest pain which may radiate to the arms, neck
and jaw. Associated with

– exercise.
– emotion.
– cold weather.
– heavy meals.
– anxiety.
– tachycardia.

Problem

Chest pain.

Actions

The following drugs may prescribed by the doctor:

• Glyceryl trinitrate is given sublinguinally to relieve
  pain. This drug lowers the blood pressure and dilates
  the coronary arteries.
• Slow-release glyceryl trinitrate is used as a prophylaxis.
  This drug is swallowed.
• Other drugs which may be prescribed include isorbide
  dinitrate and nifedine.
• Beta-receptor drugs such as propranolol and meto-
  prolol are used to reduce the rate and force of the

heart beat and so reduce the oxygen demands of the myocardium.

An electrocardiogram (ECG) is performed at rest and during exercise. Cardiac catheterization and coronary angiography may be necessary in more severe cases.

Surgery is used to treat severe angina. Coronary artery by-pass grafts using the saphenous vein are increasingly being performed with good results.

Education/Support

- Counsel the person to modify activity and to avoid stress but not so much that they become an invalid.
- Arrange for the person to be seen by a dietician for advice on how they may restrict salt and animal fat in the diet. If obese, encourage a low-calorie diet.
- Encourage the person to try and cease smoking and discuss with them other ways of avoiding stress.

Myocardial infarction

Myocardial infarction is said to have occurred when the myocardial tissue is destroyed in the regions of the heart which have become deprived of their blood supply because of a blockage within the major coronary artery or one of its branches.

Assessment

- The person may experience a sudden onset of severe chest pain which is heavy, tight, crushing or constricting, radiating to neck, jaw and arms. However, sometimes people only report a feeling of indigestion and may experience no pain.
- The skin of the person may become moist and clammy with a pallor.

- Drop in blood pressure (hypotension).
- Dyspnoea (difficulty in breathing), weakness and fainting.
- Nausea and vomiting.
- Anxiety and restlessness.
- Tachycardia or bradycardia—with cardiac arrhythmias.
- Shock.
- Cardiac failure.
- 40% of people who suffer a myocardial infarction will die from it.

Most people will go to the coronary care unit for cardiac monitoring.

Problem

Chest pain.

Action

- Assess for pain, then give prescribed analgesia.
- The doctor will have usually prescribed diamorphine 5–10 mg i.v. The effect should be monitored and the dose repeated when needed. An anti-emetic is usually given at the same time.
- Aspirin 150 mg orally immediately.
- Streptokinase 1.5 mega-units i.v. over one hour unless contraindicated. Nursing care will include care of the person receiving i.v. therapy.

Problem

Anxiety related to uncertainty and fear of dying.

Action

- Be aware that for the person it is a life-threatening situation; being in the coronary care unit can make them feel vulnerable and helpless, and they have to adjust to a change of environment.

- Answer all the questions that the person is concerned about.
- Tranquillizers, e.g. diazepam, may be prescribed. This can decrease the anxiety felt by the person.

Problem

The person may have difficulty in breathing because of the imbalance of their oxygen supply due to myocardial infarction.

Actions

- Oxygen (24–28%) via ventimask will elevate the arterial oxygen and may relieve the cardiac ischaemia.
- Assess respiratory rate. (For care of person receiving oxygen, see Chapter 7.)

Problem

Due to cardiac instability there is a risk of future myocardial infarction.

Actions

- The person will have ECG monitoring electrodes in position to monitor the heart rhythm and to confirm the clinical diagnosis of myocardial infarction.
- Explain to the person that they are able to move about the bed when attached to the monitors, and that the movements may cause bizarre patterns on the screen.
- Assess cardiac rhythm.
  Arrhythmias may be treated as follows:
  – Sinus bradycardia:
      atropine

　　　　isoprenaline
－ Atrial fibrillation:
　　　digoxin
　　　DC electroconversion
－ Heart block:
　　　atropine
　　　isoprenaline
　　　pacemaker
－ Ventricular ectopics:
　　　lignocaine
－ Ventricular fibrillation:
　　　DC electroconversion
　　　sodium bicarbonate
• Measure and record apical and radial beats, and blood pressure, at least hourly.

Problem

Pyrexia may occur 24–48 hours after a myocardial infarction. This is due to the necrosis of the myocardium.

Actions

• Record temperature frequently.
• Fan and sponge the person as necessary.

Problem

Weakness, tiredness and exhaustion.

Actions

• Person will be on complete bed-rest for 48 hours after myocardial infarction; this will help to reduce myocardial oxygen demands.
• Care must be planned to minimize interruptions of rest.

Problem

Risk of developing renal problem because of impaired blood supply to the kidney causing sodium and water retention.

Actions

- Chart fluid intake and output. Weigh daily to detect fluid overload.
- Person usually has low-cholesterol, low-salt, low-caffeine/diet. Caffeine must be limited as it is a cardiac stimulant.

Problem

Risk of constipation due to diet and bed-rest.

Actions

- Administer stool softeners and high-fibre diets.
- A commode is preferable to a bedpan. It requires less energy to use a commode, so constipation can be relieved with less myocardial demand.
- Person will gradually increase ambulation and self-care activities.

Education/Support

The person must be informed of what has happened to their heart, and health education will be planned for the individual person and their family. In some health authorities an appointment will be made for the person and family to be advised by a cardiac education nurse specialist.

HEART FAILURE

Heart failure is the heart's inability to produce a cardiac output sufficient to maintain the blood flow to the body's organs and tissues.

Failure of the left side of the heart may be the result of hypotension, aortic valve disease, myocardial infarction, mitral incompetence or mitral stenosis.

Right-sided heart failure is usually secondary to left-sided heart failure. Other causes may be myocardial infarction, affecting the right ventricle, chronic pulmonary disease, tricuspid and pulmonary valve stenosis and pericarditis.

At first the person will only have the problems of either left or right ventricular failure, but eventually the other ventricle fails because of the additional workload. The person has then developed what is termed congestive cardiac failure.

In chronic pulmonary disease the back pressure is transmitted from the lungs to the pulmonary artery, affecting the right heart and then the systemic venous circulation. The person will then have a combination of problems and any system may be involved.

Respiratory system

Problems

- Dyspnoea—laboured breathing.
- Orthopnoea—difficulty with breathing when lying flat.
- Paroxysmal nocturnal dyspnoea—this is a very frightening type of dyspnoea which awakens people from their sleep and forces them to sit up and get out of bed to catch their breath.

These problems occur because the left side of the heart is failing to pump blood forward. This causes pulmonary venous congestion, causing accumulation of fluid in the alveoli of the lungs (pulmonary oedema).

Actions

- Assist the person to sit up in a well-supported position (semi or Fowler's position) in bed or in an upright armchair. This position reduces the venous return to the heart and the lungs and alleviates pulmonary congestion and will improve chest expansion.
- Oxygen may be required via a mask/nasal cannula. (For care of the person on oxygen therapy see Chapter 7.)
- Monitor respiratory rate.

Problems

Coughing ⎫ due to congestion and fluid in
Rattling in the trachea ⎭ the alveoli which then irritates
the mucosa of the lungs

Frothy sputum. This occurs in pulmonary oedema and sometimes it may be pink coloured; this is due to the rupture of the capillaries and arterioles (pink-stained sputum is more apparent in severe congestion).

Actions

- Assist physiotherapist with encouraging the person with deep breathing exercises.
- Encourage the person with expectoration and ensure that the person has a sputum carton within reach.
- A bronchodilator, e.g. aminophylline or salbutamol, may also be prescribed to relieve bronchospasm.

Problem

Chest pain.
The person usually complains of a dull ache across the

chest. This has been caused by the congestion of the lungs and heart.

Actions

- Change in position.
- Heat pads are sometimes helpful.
- Analgesia can be used but not opiates or analgesics, which have a sedative effect.

Problem

Oedema and weight gain.
Failure of the right side of the heart leads to an increase in pressure in the great veins. This increase in venous pressure is transmitted backwards through the veins into the capillaries of the systemic circulation, resulting in a generalized oedema. Oedema can be seen in the ankles and legs but may spread to other areas such as the sacrum. It may also cause pleural effusion and ascites.

Actions

- Weight is recorded daily to monitor for the development of fluid retention.
- Position of the person is changed two-hourly; the skin is often taut and friable and may predispose to the formation of pressure sores.
- A bed cradle may be used to relieve pressure on the oedematous legs.

Problem

Reduction in urine output.
The cardiac output is insufficient to maintain the blood flow to the body organs, i.e. the kidneys.

The effect of the poor blood flow to the kidneys leads to the release of renin and the formation of angiotensin, which stimulates the adrenal cortex to release aldosterone, which causes the reabsorption of sodium by the kidneys. As a result there is a retention of sodium chloride and water. The volume of urine will decrease, and the urine will have a high specific gravity and may contain albumin.

Actions

- Assess and measure fluid output and input.
- These charts will assess the effect of diuretic drugs which may be prescribed.
- There may be fluid restriction.
- Test urine daily.

Problems

- Anorexia
- Nausea
- Vomiting

Due to enlargement of the liver, stomach and bowel

Actions

- A light well-presented diet in small quantities is offered. (Constipation can be prevented by plenty of roughage in the diet; bran or mild aperients may be helpful.)
- Nutritious drinks.
- Salt intake is restricted. (Synthetic salt may be offered as sodium restriction in the diet can sometimes be unpalatable.)
- Anti-emetics, e.g. metoclopramide, may be used to relieve nausea.

Cardiovascular

Problem

Risk of progression of cardiac failure or cardiac shock, due to heart losing its action as a pump.

Actions

Assess blood pressure and pulse frequently and decrease observations when the person's condition is stable.

Problem

Cyanosis of lips, nail beds and skin, due to reduction in peripheral blood supply.

Action

Observe the person for any changes in colour; if cyanosis develops, oxygen may help.

Problem

Risk of confusion due to insufficient oxygenation of the brain.

Actions

- Observe the person for any changes in orientation.
- Be aware of safety procedures to protect the person from injury (e.g. cot sides may be needed, and the bed lowered).
- Explain to the family the reasons why the person may be confused.
- Administration of oxygen may help to increase the oxygen levels in the circulatory blood.

Problem

Digoxin is often prescribed to improve cardiac output, so there is a risk of complications of digitalis therapy.

Actions

- Pulse and apical heart beat recordings.
- Note for slowing of pulse.
- Change in rhythm.

Problem

The person may complain of feeling cold. The skin feels cold and moist and the person may have a sub-normal temperature. This is due to the low cardiac output and inadequate circulation leading to loss of heat production.

Actions

- Evaluate temperature two-hourly.
- Keep the person warm and comfortable with bed socks, flannelette sheets, etc.

Problem

Fatigue
Exhaustion
Weakness

Due to the decreased cardiac output, the oxygen supply to the tissues is diminished.

Actions

- Rest—nursing care must be well planned to promote rest and to prevent interruptions when the person is resting.

- Assistance with activities of daily living.
- A commode is easier to use than a bedpan.

Problem

Person at risk of developing problems of bed-rest.

Action

See Chapter 3 for care of the dependent person.

Problem

Anxiety and distress due to difficulties in breathing.

Actions

- Be aware of the person's feelings, and try to avoid situations that might cause the person anxiety.
- Offer careful explanations and answers to the person's questions.
- A light on by the bed at night is reassuring for the person.

Education/Support

- The person should avoid excess in eating and drinking.
- A diet plan may be given to the person with a list of permitted and restricted foods.
- If overweight, should take a weight reduction diet until optimal weight is reached.
- The person must be given every encouragement to avoid smoking, as this causes vasoconstriction of the arteries.
- Inform and discuss with the person the effects and side-effects of the drugs.
- The amount and type of exercise should be discussed.
- Discuss with the person the problems that could occur

and how they should deal with them. The areas that the person must be aware of are:
- weight gain
- oedema of ankles, feet, abdomen
- shortness of breath
- fatigue
- palpitations
- How the person may receive support from the community services.
- To be aware of the support and information that is available from the British Heart Foundation.

COR PULMONALE

Cor pulmonale is right-sided heart failure, secondary to chronic obstructive airways disease. Chronic bronchitis, emphysema and occupational lung disease will increase the workload of the right heart.

The person will have a productive cough and severe dyspnoea in addition to the other symptoms of right-sided heart failure.

HEART BLOCK

Heart block occurs when the conducting system of the heart is impaired, resulting in failure of initiation or conduction of the electrical impulses which precede contraction of the cardiac muscle.

If there is a complete block at the atrioventricular node in the conducting system of the heart then the ventricles will beat at a rate of 30 to 40 per minute. This rate cannot maintain cardiac output and results in an inadequate blood supply to the brain, kidneys and coronary arteries. Stokes–Adams attacks are episodes of syncope caused by periods of ventricular standstill.

The treatment of complete heart block is insertion of an artificial pacemaker. This is an electronic device that delivers an electrical stimulus to the heart through a pacing wire electrode, which is inserted in or on the right ventricle.

A permanent pacemaker involves embedding the pulse generator into the subcutaneous tissue in the chest wall or upper abdominal wall. The battery will have to be changed every six to ten years.

SUBACUTE BACTERIAL ENDOCARDITIS

Subacute bacterial endocarditis is the inflammation of the endocardium caused by bacteria. It usually occurs in people who have existing valvular disease, congenital heart defects, or prosthetic valves. Vegetations of bacteria form on the valves.

The causative organism is most often *Streptococcus viridans*, which is found in infected teeth, gums and tonsils. *Streptococcus* may particularly be released into the bloodstream after dental extractions.

Assessment

Fever
Tiredness due to anaemia
Anorexia
Malaise
Weight loss
Splinter haemorrhages under the nails
Petechial haemorrhages into the skin
Painful hard lumps on fingers and toes (Osler's nodes)
Haematuria
Enlarged spleen

The person may also have a raised white cell count, and raised erythrocyte sedimentation rate (ESR).

Medical investigations

- Blood cultures are taken and the causative organism identified.
- Antibiotic therapy is commenced. Intravenous benzylpenicillin is most commonly used and large doses are given for several weeks. Oral antibiotic therapy is started when the temperature falls.

Problem

Pyrexia.

Action

For care of a person with a pyrexia see page 44.

Problem

Tiredness due to anaemia.

Actions

- Assistance given with actions of daily living.
- Person will rest in bed, only getting up to use the commode. They may be on bed-rest for a prolonged period of time, e.g. two to eight weeks.

Problem

Risk of developing problems of bed-rest.

Action

For care of the dependent person see Chapter 3.

Problem

Risk of developing complications of disease and therapy.

Action

Assess blood pressure, pulse and respirations four-hourly.

Education/Support

There is a risk of embolism from the vegetation on the endocardium of the valves; hemiplegia, renal failure, loss of vision, or ischaemia of a limb may result. Severe heart failure can also occur. Therefore, if the person is at risk it is vital that the early signs and problems of these complications are discussed with them, so that they understand how to deal with them.

Ensure:

- That the person understands the importance of carrying a card with medical information at all times.
- That when the person is receiving dental treatment, they should be having prophylactic antibiotics before and after treatment.
- That if the person develops any infection, especially respiratory, they must get it treated promptly.

PERICARDITIS

Pericarditis is inflammation of the pericardium. It may occur after acute myocardial infarction or during rheumatic fever or tuberculosis. It may also occur as a complication of other disorders, e.g. uraemia or connective tissue disorders.

Chest pain is usually present, a 'friction rub' is heard on auscultation, and a chest X-ray may show a collection of fluid in the pericardial sac. Fever is usually present. The underlying cause is treated. Indomethacin, an anti-inflammatory drug, is useful for the relief of pain.

HYPERTENSION

Raised blood pressure (hypertension) may be defined as a diastolic blood pressure persistently above 90 mmHg. Blood pressure increases with age in Western societies.

Hypertension may be primary (essential) or secondary. Primary hypertension accounts for 90% of all cases. The cause is unknown although obesity, stress and a familial tendency may be contributory factors. The major blood vessels become sclerosed and narrowed.

Secondary hypertension accounts for the remaining 10% of cases. The common causes are:

Renal disease
Endocrine disease, e.g. Cushing's disease
Cardiovascular disease, e.g. coarctation of the aorta
Hormone therapy, e.g. oral contraceptives, steroids
Drug therapy, e.g. some antidepressants
Other causes, e.g. pregnancy, raised intracranial pressure

Assessment

Sometimes hypertension may produce no problems and may only be diagnosed at a medical examination:

Headache
Vomiting
Memory impairment
Blood pressure consistently higher than 90 mmHg diastolic
Shortness of breath and angina due to increased workload on the heart
Proteinuria
– due to renal impairment
– chronic renal failure may result
Visual disturbances

– retinal haemorrhages
– oedema of the optic disc (papilloedema)

Medical investigations and during treatment

- Blood is taken for estimation of urea and electrolytes. Increased levels may indicate renal impairment.
- An intravenous urogram (see page 258) is performed.
- Diuretics are very useful for the more elderly patient.

Cyclopenthiazide with potassium (Navidrex-K) and bendrofluazide are commonly used.

- Common antihypertensive drugs include:
  beta-blockers, e.g. propranolol
  alpha-blockers, e.g. labetalol
  Vasodilators, e.g. hydralazine (prazosin)
  Others, e.g. methyldopa, captopril

Problem

Risk of developing problems as a result of underlying pathology.

Actions

- A 24-hour urine collection for vanillylmandelic acid (VMA) is normally performed in order to detect the presence of a rare tumour of the adrenal glands, a phaeochromocytoma which may cause hypertension. The person should not eat foods containing vanilla throughout the duration of this test.
- Urine tested daily for blood and protein.
- Blood pressure recorded six-hourly with the person lying and standing. (Postural hypotension may occur as a side-effect of some of the prescribed drugs.)

- Urine output recorded.
- Observe the person for any nervous system complications, e.g.
  - headaches
  - vomiting
  - difficulty with vision

Education/Support

The condition is carefully discussed with the person and family to ensure that compliancy with drug therapy will be satisfactory.

Advise the person about taking rest periods during the day and try to avoid situations that would create anxiety for them. If the person smokes they should be advised to give up. Advice is given concerning the restriction of salt and animal fats in the diet. Some people may require a low-calorie diet.

Complications of hypertension

Hypertension, if inadequately treated, may predispose to myocardial infarction, congestive cardiac failure, end-stage renal failure, cerebrovascular accident and loss of vision. Malignant hypertension is said to occur when there is severe hypertension, papilloedema, retinal haemorrhages and renal failure.

PERIPHERAL VASCULAR DISEASE

Peripheral vascular disease results in reduced circulation to the limbs, causing lack of oxygen and nutrients in the tissues. The most common cause is atherosclerosis. This condition usually affects people over the age of 50 and is more common in men. People with diabetes are particularly prone to peripheral vascular disease.

Problems

Intermittent claudication
– pain on exercise which ceases with rest
  Cold extremities
  Ulceration
  Gangrene

Arteriography may be performed to show the extent of damage to the arteries.

Actions

- Nursing actions are designed to:
  – relieve pain
  – assist rest and sleep
  – give education
- Obese people are given dietary advice.
- Animal fats should be restricted.
- Smoking should cease.
- Good control of diabetes is essential.
- The person is advised to visit a chiropodist regularly to avoid injury to the feet and to have infections treated promptly. Well-fitting shoes and socks are essential.
- Extremities of heat and cold should be avoided.

CARDIAC ARREST

Cardiac arrest is sudden failure of the heart to supply an adequate circulation. The most common causes are:

myocardial infarction
electrolyte imbalance
anaesthesia

drowning
electrocution

The heart should be restarted within three minutes to prevent irreparable damage to the brain cells due to lack of oxygen.

Problems

Loss of consciousness
Absence of major pulse
Pallor and cyanosis
Cessation of breathing
Dilation of pupils
Ventricular fibrillation or asystole on the ECG

Actions

- The lower third of the sternum is thumped with a clenched fist.
- External cardiac massage is commenced: the heel of one hand is placed over the lower third of the sternum, the heel of the other hand is placed over the first, and the sternum is depressed forcefully at a rate of about 60 times per minute.
- The airway is cleared by removing false teeth. The neck is extended and the jaw pulled forward in order to stop the tongue falling back. A plastic oral airway is inserted and mouth to mouth resuscitation is commenced at a rate of one breath to every five cardiac compressions.
- An Ambu bag may be used to ventilate the lungs.
- The nurse should be familiar with the cardiac arrest telephone and with the whereabouts of the emergency equipment.
- Relatives are escorted to a quiet room away from the activity. They should be kept informed of all developments.

Medical treatment*

- An endotracheal tube is inserted when the anaesthetist arrives.
- An intravenous infusion is set up; it is usually inserted into the subclavian or the external jugular vien.
- The following drugs may be used during a cardiac arrest:
  calcium chloride 10%
  isoprenaline
  adrenaline
  glucose (dextrose) 50%
  lignocaine 1%
  naloxone
  aminophylline
  diazepam
  frusemide
- Sodium bicarbonate 8.4% infusion may be used in a prolonged resuscitation attempt.
- DC electroconversion will be used if ventricular fibrillation is present. Everyone should stand well clear of the person and the bed to avoid getting an electric shock.

FURTHER READING

BEEVERS, G. & BEEVERS, M. (1990). Detection and assessment (hypertension). *Practice Nurse*, 2(8), 360–363.

BLACK, P. A. (1990). A preventable tragedy. The nurse's role in preventing coronary heart disease. *Professional Nurse*, 5, Issue 8, 404–410.

BARNETT, W. J. (1980). Rehabilitation for coronary care—The nurse's role. *Nursing Times*, 10 April, 20–23.

CARSON, P. (1989). Rehabilitation after myocardial infarction. *Care of the Critically Ill*, 5(5), 192–194.

CLARK MACLEOD, J., HAVERTY, S. & KENDALL, S. (1990). Helping people to stop smoking. A study of the nurse's role. *Journal of Advanced Nursing*, 16, 357–363.

FORD, J. S. (1989). Living with a history of a heart attack. A human science investigation. *Journal of Advanced Nursing*, 14, 173–179.

HOLMES, S. (1985). The Risk Business. C.O.M.A. report on diet and cardiovascular disease and the role of nurses in implementing the findings. *Senior Nurse*, **2**, No. 2,

JULIAN, D. Y. (1988). *Cardiology*, 5th edn. Baillière Tindall, London.

MAJOROWICZ, K. & HAYES CHRISTIANSEN, C. V. (1989). *Cardio-vascular Nursing*, 1st edn. W.B. Saunders, Philadelphia.

MURRAY, P. J. (1989). Rehabilitation, information and health beliefs in the post coronary patient. Do we meet their information needs? *Journal of Advanced Nursing*, **14**, 683–693.

THOMPSON, D. R. & WEBSTER, R. A. (1990). *Caring for the Coronary Patient*. Heinemann, Oxford.

7 Nursing people with problems of their respiratory system

The respiratory system allows oxygen to be absorbed into the blood and carbon dioxide to be excreted. During inspiration atmospheric air is sucked in through the nose, pharynx, larynx, trachea, bronchi, bronchioles and alveolar ducts to reach the alveoli (Figure 7.1). Oxygen then passes from the alveoli into the capillary blood, and carbon dioxide passes from the blood into the alveoli to be expired (Figure 7.2). Oxygenated blood is carried by the circulatory system to all the tissues in the body.

The following terms are used to describe abnormal functions of the respiratory system:

Dyspnoea—difficulty in breathing
Apnoea—temporary cessation of breathing
Orthopnoea—difficulty in breathing unless in an upright position
Hypoxia—reduced oxygen supply to the tissues
Cyanosis—blue discoloration of the skin or mucous membranes caused by imperfect oxygenation of the blood

NURSING ASSESSMENT OF THE PERSON WITH RESPIRATORY DISEASE

The nurse who admits a person suffering from a respiratory disorder will usually identify the first problem as breathlessness. This can result from any obstruction to breathing, especially excessive secretions, foreign

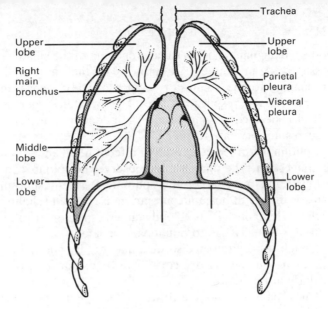

Figure 7.1 The respiratory tract.

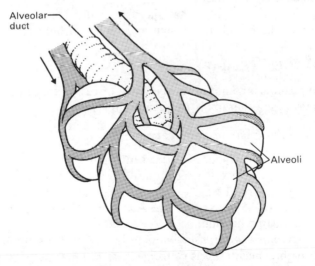

Figure 7.2 The alveoli and capillary network.

bodies, malignancy, or spasm and oedema of the small air passages. A pneumothorax, injuries of the chest wall, or damage to the respiratory centre can also cause an increase in the respiratory rate. The breathless person will also be anxious and tired. Their fear may increase their respiratory rate further.

Sputum is formed as a result of infection, inflammation or congestion. The nurse should observe the colour, consistency and quantity of the sputum. Purulent sputum consists mainly of pus; mucoid sputum is clear and slightly sticky. Haemoptysis is blood-stained sputum. Frothy sputum is usually due to pulmonary oedema.

Cough in respiratory disorders may be dry and irritating, or productive. A dry cough can be exhausting, particularly at night.

Chest pain may be due to tracheitis, when it is worse on coughing, or inflammation of the pleura, when it is greatest on inspiration.

Cyanosis indicates that there is insufficient oxygenation of the blood. It is a sign of respiratory failure.

OXYGEN THERAPY

Hypoxia is a common consequence of respiratory disease and oxygen therapy is frequently prescribed.

Methods of administration are:

1. *Ventimask* (Figure 7.3a): used when an accurate percentage of oxygen is required, especially in chronic respiratory disease. These masks can deliver 24%, 28% or 35% oxygen. They do not allow rebreathing of carbon dioxide.
2. *MC mask or Hudson mask* (Figure 7.3b): used when high concentrations of oxygen are required, e.g. 35 to 65%. Rebreathing of carbon dioxide occurs.
3. *Nasal cannulae* (Figure 7.3c): these allow the person to

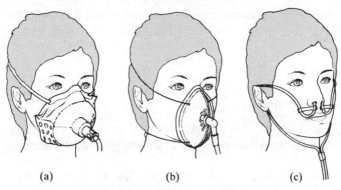

(a)   (b)   (c)

Figure 7.3 Methods of administering supplemental oxygen to the intubated person. (a) A Ventimask. (b) A MC or Hudson mask. (c) Nasal cannulae.

    eat and drink normally, and to communicate easily. The concentration of oxygen may vary.
4. *Oxygen tents*: used for young children.
5. *Head boxes*: useful for infants and young children.
6. *Ventilators*: can be operated with air or oxygen. A range of concentrations can be used.

    The mouth and nose can become very dry during oxygen therapy. Fluids are encouraged and mouth care performed. These people often appreciate ice to suck. Humidification is necessary with high concentrations of oxygen.

    In chronic obstructive airways disease, sensitivity of the respiratory centre to carbon dioxide is impaired and the person relies on the hypoxic drive to maintain respiration. If too high a concentration of oxygen is given, carbon dioxide retention will occur and respiration will be depressed. The nurse should observe these people continuously for signs of respiratory depression.

    Oxygen in excess is toxic to the lining of the bronchi and alveoli, eventually leading to gross stiffness of the lungs and hypoxia.

Oxygen supports combustion, so smoking should be prohibited in an area where oxygen is being used.

INVESTIGATIONS

Lung function tests

Vital capacity is the largest volume of air which can be expelled from the lungs after full inspiration. It measures loss of lung volume.

Peak expiratory flow rate (PEFR) is the maximum flow, in litres per minute, at the beginning of forced expiration from full inspiration. It is measured using a peak flow meter, and measures airflow obstruction.

Arterial blood gases measure gas transfer from the air to the blood.

Radiography

The person with a respiratory problem will have an X-ray of the chest. Tomograms illustrate the depth of lesions in the lung. Screening can be used to determine the position and function of the diaphragm.

A bronchogram is the introduction of dye into the lungs to outline the walls of the bronchi. Radioisotope scanning may be performed, and is of special value when pulmonary emboli are suspected.

Bronchoscopy

A flexible fibreoptic bronchoscope is used to inspect the trachea and larger bronchi (Figure 7.4). Tissue can be removed (a biopsy) for examination. This procedure is usually performed under local anaesthesia. A rigid bronchoscope is used for removal of foreign bodies or copious secretions.

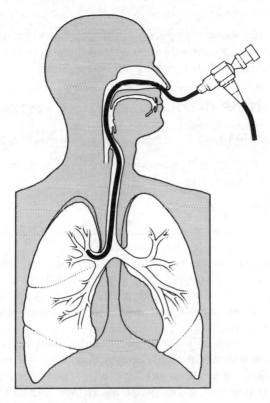

Figure 7.4 Fibreoptic bronchoscopy.

After bronchoscopy the person must have nothing to eat or drink until the cough reflex has returned.

Laryngoscopy

Indirect laryngoscopy is inspection of the larynx using a small mirror placed at the back of the mouth. Direct laryngoscopy is inspection of the larynx using a laryngoscope.

Mediastinoscopy

Mediastinoscopy is inspection of the mediastinum using a fibreoptic endoscope through a small incision in the chest wall. Enlarged lymph nodes can be biopsied.

INFECTIONS OF THE RESPIRATORY SYSTEM

Acute bronchitis

This is an acute inflammation of the mucous membranes of the bronchial tree.

Predisposing causes

- Can be caused by bacteria, such as *Streptococcus pneumoniae* and *Haemophilus influenzae*.
- Complication of the common cold, influenza, measles, or whooping cough.
- Can also be caused by dust and smoke. As air pollution increases, so too does the incidence of acute bronchitis.
- More common in the winter months when people are exposed to damp, cold, or foggy conditions. Cigarette smoking may also predispose to acute bronchitis. Bronchitis can affect people of all ages but is usually only dangerous to the old and the very young and those weakened by some other disease.

Assessment

Cough
– dry and irritating at first
– productive later
Chest pain
– retrosternal pain due to tracheitis
Sputum

– mucopurulent
– sometimes streaked with blood
Fever
– low-grade pyrexia
In severe cases temperature may rise to 38–39°C and
  cyanosis may be present.

Problem

Acute breathlessness and productive cough.

Actions

- Assist the person to sit upright in bed with their back
  well supported with back rest and pillows.
- A cough mixture based on codeine may be prescribed
  by the doctor which will suppress the cough and help in
  allowing the person to rest.
- Assist the physiotherapist in encouraging the person to
  cough in order to expectorate sputum.
- Put disposable sputum pot and tissues within reach
  of the person.
- Observe for changes in the amount and character of
  sputum.

Problem

Chest infection—therefore potential for deterioration
of condition.

Actions

- Monitor temperature, pulse and respirations at least
  six-hourly.
- Sputum specimen must be taken for microbiological
  examination.

- If antibiotics are prescribed they must be given on time to maintain correct blood levels.
- Aspirin may be given to reduce fever.
- Be alert for signs of exhaustion and respiratory depression.
- Observe for signs of cyanosis.

Problem

The person may be anxious and frightened about their condition.

Actions

- Understand that the constant shortness of breath and fatigue makes the person irritable and depressed.
- Be sensitive to fears and anxiety, show that you care and give clear explanations when nursing care is given. This helps to reduce a fast respiratory rate.

Problem

The person may finding it difficult to deal with activities of daily living.

Action

Assist as necessary during the acute phase.

Problem

Potential for dehydration.

Action

Encourage fluid intake of three litres daily (a good fluid intake will also decrease the viscosity of sputum and aid expectoration).

Education/Support

- Person is advised to try and stop smoking.
- Poor housing conditions may need to be investigated by the social worker.

Bronchiectasis

This is a chronic condition of the bronchi and the bronchioles with impaired drainage of bronchial secretions. There is persistent infection in the affected lobe or segment. The incidence of this condition has fallen as a result of effective antibiotic therapy.

Predisposing causes

Bronchial obstruction
- mucous plugs
- tumours
- foreign bodies
- congenital disorders
- cystic fibrosis
- obstruction by viscid sputum

Assessment

Chronic cough
Sputum
- purulent and copious
- worse in the morning
- haemoptysis common
Dyspnoea
- only present when bronchiectasis is bilateral
Sinusitis
Systemic symptoms
- weight loss and anorexia
- fever

Finger clubbing
These problems usually begin in childhood.

Problem

Breathlessness with productive cough.

Actions

• Postural drainage of the affected lobe is essential and a
  member of the family should be taught how to percuss
  the chest.
• The breathless person may prefer to sit upright in bed
  in order to sleep.
• Sputum specimens are taken for microbiological culture
  and sensitivity.
• Infections are treated promptly with antibiotics.
• Coughing and deep breathing exercises are encouraged,
  particularly on rising in the morning.
• A good fluid intake is essential in order to reduce the
  viscosity of the sputum and so aid expectoration.

Surgical intervention, e.g. removal of a lobe of the lung,
may be necessary. However, antibiotic therapy has improved the prognosis and complications are rare.

Pneumonia

Pneumonia is inflammation of the lung. Exudates of fluid,
protein and red blood cells cause consolidation of the
inflamed area.
    There are two main groups:

1. Lobar pneumonia—an acute primary infection, occurring in a previously healthy respiratory tract. The
   whole of the lobe becomes consolidated.
2. Bronchopneumonia—infected material is aspirated

from the upper respiratory tract. Patches of inflammation are scattered in one lobe, several lobes or over both lungs. Bronchopneumonia commonly occurs secondary to other conditions such as chronic bronchitis or carcinoma of the bronchus.

Predisposing causes

Pneumonia is usually caused by bacteria. Common organisms causing lobar pneumonia are:

Streptococcus pneumoniae (pneumococcus)
Streptococcus pyogenes
Klebsiella pneumoniae
Mycoplasma pneumoniae

Viruses may also be responsible for lobar pneumonia.
Common organisms causing bronchopneumonia are:

Streptococcus pneumoniae
Staphylococcus aureus
Haemophilus influenzae

Predisposing causes of pneumonia are:

Viral infections
– influenza
– measles
– chickenpox
Chronic obstructive airways disease
Bronchial obstruction
– tumours
– foreign bodies
– retention of secretions (especially following anaesthesia)
Aspiration
– unconsciousness
– oesophageal fistula
– motor neurone disease

Impaired resistance
- steroid or cytotoxic therapy
- elderly
- malnutrition
- very young
- diabetes mellitus
- chronic renal failure

There is a high-risk mortality rate in bronchopneumonia, especially in the very young and the old. Early treatment of respiratory infections is essential.

Assessment

Fever
- 38–40°C
- causes rigors
Systemic disturbances
- vomiting
Confusion
- especially in the elderly
- due to hypoxia
Respiratory problems
- dyspnoea
- rapid respiratory rate
- pleuritic chest pain
- cough
- cyanosis
- sputum
Cardiovascular problems
- tachycardia
- atrial fibrillation and heart failure in the young and old
- hypotension due to dehydration and infection
Herpes simplex
- around the mouth and lips
- in lobar pneumonia

Medical investigations

- Oxygen therapy may be prescribed if the person is hypoxic.
- Antibiotics will be prescribed. They may be given orally or intravenously.
- Intravenous fluids may be necessary if severe dehydration is present.
- Mild analgesics, e.g. paracetamol or aspirin, are prescribed to relieve the chest pain.
- Bronchodilator drugs, e.g. salbutamol, are given in more severe cases.

Problems

- Difficulty in breathing/wheezing.
- Risk of respiratory distress/deterioration.

Actions

- Assist the person to sit upright in bed, and position the arms comfortably away from the chest to avoid them restricting chest movements.
- Record vital signs as condition warrants.
  - respiratory rate.
  - observe for pallor, cyanosis.
  - pulse rate, observe for tachycardia and alteration in rhythm.
  - Note nature and frequency of coughing, difficult expectoration, haemoptysis.
- Oxygen may be ordered. It can be administered by mask or nasal cannula. The method used will depend on the person's condition and oxygen requirements. (For care of a person receiving oxygen therapy see page 124.)
- Assist the physiotherapist with intensive physiotherapy;

this will help with chest expansion and expectoration of the sputum.

- Turn the person two-hourly to facilitate removal of secretions from the lungs.
- Provide a disposable sputum pot and paper tissues within reach of the person.
- Adjust the care plan of the person so that after physio-therapy sessions they will be able to rest before other procedures are carried out.

Problem

Risk of the person becoming dehydrated due to sweating and rapid respiratory rate.

Actions

- Encourage fluid intake, two to three litres daily.
- Record intake and output.
- Frequent mouth care would be appreciated by the person.
- Observe for confusion and increased restlessness which may occur as a result of severe dehydration.
- The person may require intravenous therapy.

Problem

Risk of developing problems of bed-rest.
Actions.
See Chapter 3.

Education/Support

Pneumonia can be very debilitating, so the person should be advised to rest as much as possible. Elderly people may require a long stay in hospital before they are fully recovered.

Pulmonary tuberculosis

Pulmonary tuberculosis is a disease caused by the micro-organism *Mycobacterium tuberculosis*. The human type of the mycobacterium is commonly responsible for the disease in man.

Bovine tuberculosis has been eradicated in the United Kingdom as a result of the pasteurization of milk and the veterinary inspection of cattle.

Most tuberculosis infections are due to the inhalation of air containing the tubercle bacilli, coughed up by an infectious person.

An area of inflammation occurs in the alveoli (primary focus) and the lymph nodes in the hilum of the lung enlarge. This infection usually resolves unnoticed. Failure to resolve will result in an area of caseation (cheese-like consistency), and fibrosis and calcification may occur, resulting in lung cavities. Pleural effusion, haemoptysis and pneumothorax may result.

Miliary tuberculosis occurs when the tubercle bacilli spread into the bloodstream, and tuberculosis of bones, joints and the genitourinary tract may occur. Tuberculosis meningitis may also accompany this condition.

Predisposing factors

Tuberculosis is most commonly seen in the underdeveloped countries. Although tuberculosis is not as prevalent in the United Kingdom as it was, there is an increase in people suffering from this problem associated with those who have come to this country from areas where tuberculosis is more common.

Tuberculosis is associated with overcrowded housing, poor nutrition and alcoholism. It is more common in males over the age of 45 years.

People with the following conditions are susceptible to tuberculosis.

- Diabetes.
- Having steroid or immunosuppressive therapy.
- With congenital heart disease.
- Have had a gastrectomy.

Assessment

Uncomplicated primary infection may be free of problems.

Fever
- night sweats
- anorexia and weight loss
- weakness due to anaemia
- pleuritic pain
Hoarseness
- due to laryngitis
Cough
- usually productive
- haemoptysis
Dyspnoea

Medical treatment

The main treatment of pulmonary tuberculosis is drug therapy.

- Treatment with anti-tuberculosis drugs can last 18 months to 2 years. Three anti-tuberculosis drugs are given at first; this is known as 'triple therapy'. Three drugs are used as resistance can quickly develop if only one is used. The most commonly used drugs are:
  Rifampicin (400–600 mg daily)
  - colours the urine red
  Isoniazid (200–300 mg daily)
  - may cause peripheral neuritis
  - pyridoxine (vitamin B_6) 10 mg often given prophy-lactically.
  Ethambutol (15 mg/kg daily)
  - may cause optic neuritis

- In underdeveloped countries, streptomycin and isoniazid are used on two days/week.
- People with pulmonary tuberculosis will require standard isolation nursing (see Chapter 4).

Education/Support

The person is discharged from hospital when their sputum is no longer infectious. They are advised to comply with their drug therapy and to attend their out-patient appointment.

OCCUPATIONAL LUNG DISEASES

The most common occupational lung diseases are those caused by the inhalation of mineral dusts (pneumoconiosis). Fibrosis of the lung can occur, resulting in progressive breathlessness, respiratory failure and cardiac failure. The most common types of pneumoconiosis are:

coal worker's pneumoconiosis
silicosis
asbestosis

Silicosis can predispose to pulmonary tuberculosis. Asbestosis can predispose to malignant disease of the pleura and peritoneum.

The Department of Social Security provide compensation for those workers affected by occupational lung diseases. Prevention, however, is very important. Industries are obliged by law to ensure that their workers use respirators where necessary. Adequate ventilation and damping down of coal is essential.

CHRONIC OBSTRUCTIVE AIRWAYS DISEASE

Chronic bronchitis and emphysema often coexist and are grouped together under the term 'chronic obstructive airways disease'. Chronic bronchitis is chronic inflammation of the lung due to long-term exposure of the bronchial mucosa to irritants. Emphysema is the enlargement of the alveoli and the destruction of their walls. The lungs become overdistended and lose their normal elasticity.

Chronic obstructive airways disease is more common in middle-aged and elderly men.

Predisposing causes

The common irritants which cause chronic bronchitis are tobacco smoke, dust, fumes and smoke. Infection aggravates the condition and is usually due to the bacteria *Streptococcus pneumoniae* or *Haemophilus influenzae*.

This condition is usually worse during the winter months, especially after exposure to dampness, fog or a change in temperature.

Assessment

Cough
- repeated attacks of a productive 'winter cough'
- usually worse in the morning
Sputum
- sometimes scanty, mucoid and tenacious
- sometimes copious and watery
- purulent if bacterial infection is present
Dyspnoea
- worse on exertion
- caused by airways obstruction
- aggravated by infection and mucosal oedema
Barrel-shaped, rigid chest (in emphysema)
Cyanosis
- worse on exertion
Peripheral oedema
- due to right-sided heart failure (cor pulmonale)

Problem

Shortness of breath which varies on a daily basis with usual activity, increased effort and during sleep.

Actions

- Understand that the constant shortness of breath and fatigue makes the person irritable, anxious and depressed.
- Be sensitive to the person's fears and anxiety. Show that you care and give clear explanations when nursing care is given.
- Oxygen at 24–28% via a Ventimask is prescribed (see page 124).
- The person is assisted to sit upright with their back well supported with back rest and pillows. Sometimes the person may feel more comfortable in a high-backed chair.
- The person will require intensive physiotherapy. Assist the person to cough and expectorate.
- Check that a sputum pot and disposable tissues are within reach of the person.
- Bronchodilator drugs, e.g. salbutamol, can be given by inhalation, tablet form or intravenously.
- Aminophylline, another bronchodilator, is especially useful when given in suppository form prior to the person settling for the night.
- Peak flow readings should be taken before and 20 minutes after bronchodilator drugs are given.
- Hypnotics and sedatives are avoided because they may lead to respiratory depression.

Problem

Risk of developing a chest infection.

Actions

- Temperature and pulse are recorded at least six-hourly.
- Sputum specimens are taken for microbiological examination.
- Antibiotics, e.g. amoxycillin, may be used to treat the chest infection.
- Respiratory rate, level of consciousness and colour should be observed carefully when the person is receiving oxygen. (For care of person receiving oxygen therapy see page 124).

Problem

Risk of becoming dehydrated.

Actions

- Encourage fluid intake of two to three litres in 24 hours; this will also aid expectoration of sputum.
- Frequent mouth care would be appreciated by the person.

Problem

Risk of peripheral oedema developing due to right-sided heart failure (cor pulmonale).

Actions

- Blood pressure should be recorded six-hourly.
- Weigh daily in order to monitor the effect of any diuretic used.

Problem

At risk of developing the complications of bed-rest.

Actions

See Chapter 3.

Education/Support

A clear explanation should be given to the person of what to expect and how to live with their problems:

- Avoid exposure to certain environments, e.g. where there is smoke, dust, fumes, or people who may be suffering from respiratory infections.
- Understand that any respiratory infection must be treated promptly, and prescribed antibiotics, must be taken.
- Maintain an adequate fluid intake; this will help to reduce the viscosity of the sputum and so aid expectoration.
- Understand the importance of continuing breathing exercises which strengthen the muscles of expiration and so empty the lungs more fully.
- Maintain general health at the best possible level.

Chronic obstructive airways disease can be very disabling. Premature retirement may be necessary, resulting in socio-economic problems. The person may eventually become housebound, often relying on oxygen to move from room to room. The person might also need the support of the community services such as a home-help and meals-on-wheels. Britain has the highest mortality rate from bronchitis.

BRONCHIAL CARCINOMA

Carcinoma of the bronchus is the most common primary neoplasm in men in Britain. It is a disease of middle and old age. The incidence among women is increasing.

Causes

The incidence of bronchial carcinoma is higher in cigarette smokers and those living in urban areas. Workers who are exposed to asbestos, nickel and radioactive substances have an increased risk of bronchial carcinoma. Carcinoma of the bronchus can be treated by surgery, radiotherapy, chemotherapy, or a combination of these. Surgical treatment consists of a lobectomy (removal of a lobe) or pneumonectomy (removal of a lung).

Assessment

Cough
Sputum
– sometimes bloodstained
– sometimes purulent
   because of secondary infection

Systemic disturbances
– weight loss
– anorexia
– weakness
– dysphagia
– hoarseness

Chest pain
Breathlessness
– rarely disabling
Problems due to metastic deposits
– e.g. bone pain or hemiplegia

The problems and needs of a person with carcinoma are discussed in Chapter 5.

Conclusion

The prognosis of carcinoma of the bronchus is poor. Of those who have had surgery, 25 to 30% survive five years; however, surgery is only feasible for 25% of cases. The person and their family will need much support from their general practitioner, district nurse and social worker. The hospice movement is expanding, and in many areas a terminal care support team is available to look after these people in their own homes.

The risk of developing carcinoma of the bronchus can be reduced by a reduction in cigarette smoking. Protective clothing should be worn by workers who are exposed to carcinogenic substances.

ASTHMA

Bronchial asthma is a temporary narrowing of the bronchi by muscle spasm and mucosal oedema. Air becomes trapped in the alveoli. It is characterized by attacks of dyspnoea and wheezing.

Types of asthma

1. Extrinsic asthma occurs in people who are allergic to common allergens, including house dust, mites, grass, pollen, fur and feathers. There is usually a family history of allergic disease, especially eczema and hay fever. These individuals are described as being 'atopic'.
2. Intrinsic asthma occurs in non-atopic individuals in later life. There is no obvious allergic factor.
3. The problems of asthma can be precipitated by exposure to dust, tobacco smoke, fumes, infections and stress.

Assessment

Dyspnoea
– attacks of dyspnoea and wheezing
– wheeze is more pronounced on expiration
– accessory muscles are used to aid expiration
– exhaustion can lead to respiratory failure
Cyanosis
– the face becomes congested
– extremities are cyanosed
Tachycardia
– present in severe attacks

Sputum
- scanty at first
- sometimes viscid

Stress

Status asthmaticus
- severe, worsening asthma
- eventually leads to:
  exhausation and inability to cough
  cyanosis
  disturbances of consciousness
  respiratory failure

Problem

Attacks of dyspnoea and wheezing.

Actions

- Oxygen is prescribed and usually administered via an MC mask. (For care of person receiving oxygen therapy see page 124.)
- Assist the person to sit upright in bed and position the arms comfortably away from the chest to avoid them restricting chest movement.
- Salbutamol, a bronchodilator, can be given by inhaler or nebulizer. In more severe cases, another bronchodilator, aminophylline (250–500 mg), can be given intravenously.
- Check respiratory rate, level of consciousness and colour of face. Note if the person is more comfortable and is beginning to relax.
- Temperature, pulse and blood pressure are taken half-hourly to four-hourly depending on the severity of the attack.

Problem

The person is frightened and anxious.

Actions

- Never leave a person during an asthmatic attack; they will need constant attention and assurance.
- Assist the physiotherapist with intensive physiotherapy; this will help with chest expansion and loosening and expectoration of the sputum.
- Sputum specimens are taken for microbiological examination.
- Steroids are given to reduce oedema of the mucosa, e.g. hydrocortisone (100–200 mg six-hourly). The dose of steroids is reduced slowly when the person's condition has stabilized.
- Urine is tested daily for sugar because of the risk of steroid-induced diabetes.
- Antibiotics, e.g. amoxycillin, are used to treat the underlying respiratory infection. They may be given orally or intravenously.
- Hypnotics and sedatives are avoided because of the risk of steroid-induced diabetes.
- Peak flow readings are taken in order to monitor the response to the bronchodilator drugs which may be prescribed.

Problem

Will need assistance with comfort and activities of daily living during and after an attack.

Action

Helping the person with washing of face and hands and changing of bed clothes is appreciated.

Problem

Risk of collapse due to exhaustion or failure to respond to treatment.

Actions

- Temperature, pulse, blood pressure are recorded half-hourly to four-hourly depending on the severity of the attack.
- Dehydration is corrected using intravenous fluids.
- After any dehydration is corrected a good fluid intake of two to three litres in 24 hours will decrease the viscosity of the sputum and so aid expectoration.
- Blood gases should be taken to monitor oxygen requirements.
- The person may require assisted ventilation.

Education/Support

The person is advised to avoid causative allergens. Respiratory infections should be treated promptly. Stressful situations should be avoided as they may precipitate an attack.

Salbutamol is given using an inhaler or Rotocaps. A Rotahaler can be used by the person during an asthmatic attack. Steroids can be given in the form of a beclomethasone inhaler. Sodium cromoglycate (Intal), given via an inhaler, prevents release of agents which cause bronchoconstriction and is used prophylactically.

Conclusion

The causative allergens can sometimes be identified by patch tests and should then be avoided if possible. It is essential to live as normal a life as possible; relatives can often become very protective towards a child with asthma.

Many children with asthma will be problem-free by the age of 15 years.

DISORDERS OF THE PLEURA

Pneumothorax

A pneumothorax is a collection of air in the pleural space causing collapse of the associated lung.

Predisposing causes

A spontaneous pneumothorax occurs when a sac of air in the lung (a bulla) ruptures through the surface of the

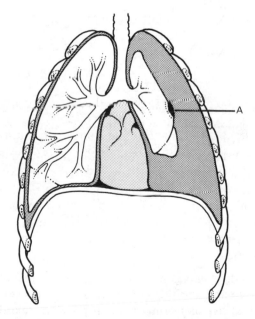

Figure 7.5   Closed pneumothorax.

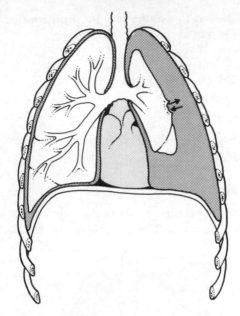

Figure 7.6 Open pneumothorax.

visceral pleura, allowing air to escape into the pleural space. Spontaneous pneumothorax mainly occurs in healthy people, especially tall young men, and is often recurrent. People with chronic bronchitis and emphysema are also susceptible to the large air sacs that may develop in the lungs in these conditions.

A pneumothorax can also be caused by penetrating wounds of the chest wall and by rib fractures. If blood is also present in the pleural space, the condition is known as haemopneumothorax.

Types

1. Closed pneumothorax (Figure 7.5). The hole between the lung and the pleural space (marked A on Figure

7.5) closes off and the air in the pleural cavity is gradually absorbed, allowing the lung to re-expand.

2. Open pneumothorax (Figure 7.6). The hole between the lung and the pleural space remains open and the lung thus remains deflated. Sometimes a direct communication between the bronchus and the pleural space can develop; this is known as a bronchopleural fistula.

3. Tension pneumothorax (Figure 7.7). The hole between the lung and the pleural space is small and acts as a one-way valve, allowing air to enter the pleural space but preventing it from escaping. The pressure in the pleural space builds up until it is above atmospheric pressure. This causes collapse of the affected lung, shift

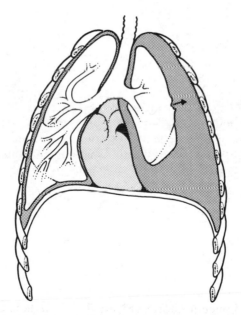

Figure 7.7   Tension pneumothorax.

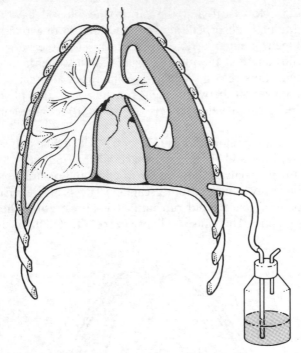

Figure 7.8 Underwater seal drainage.

of mediastinal structures, and consequent compression
of the opposite lung.

Assessment

Chest pain or tightness
Breathlessness (can rapidly worsen in a tension pneu-
    mothorax)
Cyanosis
– present in tension pneumothorax
– fatal respiratory failure can occur
Anxiety

Medical treatment

- If the pneumothorax is large an intercostal drain will be inserted into the pleural space. This is connected to an underwater seal drain (Figure 7.8). The 'water seal' allows air to leave the pleural space but prevents it from returning.
- Thoracic suction is sometimes necessary if re-expansion does not occur.
- Pain and anxiety relief is usually instantaneous, once the thoracic catheter has been introduced.

Points to be considered in caring for a person who has underwater seal drainage are as follows:

- The lower end of the tube should always be covered by the water in the drain bottle.
- The bottle should never be raised above the level of the tube insertion or water will enter the pleural space.
- The nurse ensures that the level in the tube is 'swinging' with respirations, i.e. that it is not obstructed.
- The drainage tube is clamped when the bottle is changed. If it is accidently left unclamped, a tension pneumothorax may occur because of accumulation of air in the pleural space.
- If blood is present in the tube, from trauma, 'milking' may be necessary by using a pair of rollers to prevent obstruction of the tube by blood clots.
- The person can move around, providing the drain is held below waist level.
- The thoracic catheter is removed after five to six days.
- Small pneumothoraces often resolve without intervention. Recurrent pneumothoraces can be treated surgically by performing a parietal pleurectomy (stripping of part of the parietal pleura).

Pleural effusion

A pleural effusion is a collection of fluid in the pleural space. The commonest causes are pneumonia, malignancy and tuberculosis. Transudates of fluid into the pleural space also occur in cardiac failure, renal failure, liver disease, and malnutrition. The main problem is dyspnoea.

Pleural aspiration is performed for diagnosis or treatment.

FURTHER READING

BOYLAN, A. & BROWN, P. (1985). Students' observations (respirations). *Nursing Times*, **81**, 35–38.

DURIE, M. (1984). Respiratory problems and nursing interventions. *Nursing* **2**, No. 28, 826–828.

KERSTON, L. (1989). *Comprehensive Respiratory Nursing. A Decision-Making Approach*, 1st edn. W.B. Saunders, London.

MCMILLAN, E. (1984). Oxygen therapy. *Nursing*, **2**, No. 28, 822–825.

PEARSON, R. & BARNES, G. (1989). Tests of lung function (Asthma). *Practise Nurse*, **2**(7), 315–318.

THOMPSON, M. C. (1984). Physiotherapy essentials of chest care. *Nursing*, **2**, No. 27, 796–800.

WALSH, M. (1989). Making sense of chest drainage. *Nursing Times*, **85**, No. 24, 40–41.

WILSON, S. F. & THOMPSON, J. M. (1990). *Nursing Care of Patients with Respiratory Disorders*. Mosby's Nursing Care Series, Vol. 2. C.V. Mosby, London.

8 Nursing people with problems due to cancer

The word cancer can cause fear, anxiety, pain and anguish for people and their families. These feelings are not helped by the confusion and misunderstanding that can arise from the plethora of words that are used. A vocabulary of terms has arisen which include words such as: cancer, carcinoma, tumour, growths, neoplasms, malignant, benign, metastases and secondaries.

Perhaps some of this misunderstanding arises because cancer is sometimes thought of as a specific disease. In fact it is a group of diseases and one form of cancer may have little in common with another.

Nurses need to be aware of what is meant by the term cancer, the education we can give to lessen the risk of developing types of cancer, the problems that may result if a person does develop one of these diseases, the care they will require due to these problems and the nursing intervention required as a result of surgery, radiotherapy and chemotherapy. It is also important that nurses understand the philosophy and approach behind complementary approaches to caring for people and their families as a result of this group of diseases. This understanding will help us to provide care with knowledge, empathy and skill.

This chapter will consider:

- The nature of cancers.
- The incidence of cancers.

- Causative factors of cancers.
- Early detection and prevention of cancers.
- Caring for people and their families who develop cancer.
- The nursing intervention required for people undergoing surgery, radiotherapy and chemotherapy.
- Complementary approaches to people with cancers.

THE NATURE OF CANCER

All cells of the body have the same basic structure of a nucleus enclosed by a nuclear membrane surrounded by cytoplasm, which, in turn, is surrounded by a thin cell membrane. Although the nucleus is roughly spherical, the shape of the surrounding cytoplasm can vary greatly, which gives rise to cuboidal, columnar, pyramidal or squamous cells. Within each nucleus an enormous amount of information is coded on the deoxyribonucleic acid (DNA). Long strands of DNA are coiled up to form chromosomes. This information is transmitted from the nucleus to the cytoplasm by a particular type of ribonucleic acid (RNA) which is termed a messenger RNA.

When it is necessary for more cells to be produced, the cytoplasm and nucleus will divide to produce two identical cells. This is called mitosis. In order for cell division to occur, the cell must go through a complex sequence of events prior to and in preparation for this division. This production of new cells normally occurs, or is regulated by, a process which allows for growth in early life and the replacement of worn-out or damaged cells throughout life.

Cancerous cells

If the control mechanism for the reproduction of cells is lost in a particular area of the body, then an excessive number of cells may be produced. These new cells may form an abnormal mass of tissue. This is then referred to as a new growth or a neoplasm. These cells may reproduce rapidly and change in structure and activity in a variety of ways. They serve no useful purpose.

Firstly, they alter the balance by which the cells within an organ are lost and recreated, so that the production of normal cells is disturbed. Secondly, they use nutrients and oxygen, thereby causing deprivation of the normal tissue within that part of the body. Thirdly, they may form a mass of tissue which extends beyond the confines of the organ in which they originate.

Malignant neoplasm

This term refers to situations where cancerous cells have extended outside the organ in which they started. As a result they may disturb the functions of more than the original organ and may then be carried by the blood or lymph to distant parts of the body. They may then set up colonies of these malignant cells in parts of the body far away from where they started. This is referred to as metastases or secondary spread.

Certain parts of the body are known to be the most common sites for the spread of malignant cells from one organ to another. For example, cancer cells of the stomach may spread to the liver and cancer cells of the breast may spread to the lungs, brain and bones.

Some malignant growths are graded according to the degree of differentiation of the cancerous cells and the estimated rate of growth of the mass of cells or tumour. In addition, the term staging may be used. This may be done to determine what form of medical/pharmacological intervention should be chosen. This system is sometimes referred to as TNM: T denotes the size of the tumour;

N refers to the extent of regional lymph gland involvement; and M relates to the extent of metastases.

Benign neoplasm

This term refers to a situation whereby cancerous cells
have developed but do not spread to other sites of the
body. The growth of these cells therefore tends to be slow.
They often expand within an organ and may form a
capsule round them within that organ. The cells may show
only slight differences compared to the normal cells within
that organ.

They are not therefore usually a threat to life and are
usually removed by surgery. If they are not removed they
may become malignant. Examples are polyps in the colon
and pigmented moles.

To summarize, cancerous cells have certain well-
known characteristics. In the early stages they resemble
the original cell from which they developed. With the
growth in numbers of cancerous cells they then start to
differ markedly from the original cell. These cells have the
ability to infiltrate into the tissues and spread throughout
the body. They may then cause those parts of the
body to fail to work normally and death can occur.

The term oncology refers to all new growths, whether
they are malignant or benign.

THE INCIDENCE OF CANCERS

It is estimated that approximately 25% of people in the
United Kingdom will develop cancer. However, many
people do not die from cancer. Whether death from
cancer occurs is dependent on where in the body the
cancer is and whether metastases develop. It is, though,

the second largest cause of death, circulatory disease being the first, or major cause. Of all cancers, lung cancer in men, and breast cancer in women, have the highest incidence in the United Kingdom.

The pattern of which cancers occur most commonly varies from country to country. The statistics of the incidence of certain types of cancers may provide clues as to predisposing factors: such as factors in the environment, occupational risks, habits and customs. Health education and preventative measures can then be orientated appropriately. These changing patterns from one country to another are not a function of race. If people from one country emigrate to another, then their patterns of incidence of cancer alter to that of the population in which they now live.

The incidence of cancers is influenced by:

- People living longer—the incidence of cancer increases with age.
- Greater exposure to substances which predispose a person (carcinogens) to cancer, e.g. cigarette smoke.
- New and improved diagnostic techniques.
- Decrease in deaths from other diseases such as pneumonias and other acute infections.

Although the incidence of cancer has increased, so too has the survival rate of people diagnosed as having a form of cancer. Survival rates vary considerably according to where and what form of cancer a person has. Increased survival is due to combination of better treatment/ management and earlier diagnosis of cancers.

CAUSATIVE FACTORS OF CANCER

Cancer is a diverse group of diseases and research is aimed at looking for causes of individual cancers and not at a single cause or single cure. Indeed, research is designed to identify the separate links in a whole chain of interacting causes. These links may interact over a broad time scale, such as 30 years, before the problems resulting from cancer occur.

Whatever the tissue from which cancerous cells develop, the common link is thought to be the genetic material deoxyribonucleic acid (DNA), which makes up part of the chromosomes in the nuclei of human cells. This is affected by two broad sets of factors which are both intrinsic and extrinsic. These factors which cause malignant change are known as carcinogens.

Intrinsic factors

Genetic factors

It is known that certain genetic changes make it more likely that an individual will develop cancer. This has been shown where chromosomal disorders, which involve the absence, duplication or rearrangement of genetic material, make cancer more likely. For example, people with Down's syndrome, where each cell contains an extra chromosome, are 11 times more likely to develop leukaemia.

Research is also looking at how oncogenes, which have the potential to cause cancer, when activated, and how moveable genes, which may activate the oncogene by disruption of DNA, are linked to the causation of cancers.

Hormonal factors

Certain cancers appear to be influenced by the presence of an excessive concentration of particular hormones. It is perhaps not the hormones themselves, but whether they produce tissue that is susceptible to certain cancers, that is the focus of study. This interest arises from the striking differences that exist between cancers in men and women. It has also been of interest since certain hormones started to be used in the management of some types of cancer.

Immunological factors

Research is also designed to identify the role our immune systems play in the development, suppression and progression of certain cancers. It is thought that abnormal cells of a neoplasm contain substances that are foreign (antigens) to the normal body cells. These antigens may prompt an immune response in a person's body, so that spontaneous regression and disappearance of cancerous cells occurs. In other words, we may always be developing cancerous cells, but the body is able to destroy them. Therefore research is considering whether, in certain people, their immune systems fail, and so cancerous cells then multiply. This may account for the high incidence of cancer in people with immune deficiency problems, or who are taking immune suppressing drugs, or who are exposed to radiation, or where the ageing process may make the immune system less efficient.

Extrinsic factors

Three main groups of extrinsic factors are considered predisposing to the developments of cancer: chemical agents, physical agents and viruses.

Chemical agents

Many different chemical agents have been studied as possible carcinogens and a number have been identified as known predisposing causes of cancer. Examples of these are:

- Cigarette smoking (cancers of the respiratory and urinary systems).
- Aniline dyes—absorbed through the skin (cancers of the urinary system).
- Air pollutants, e.g. asbestos (respiratory cancers).

Other chemicals such as hydrocarbons, chromates, arsenic and nickel are also suspect. Research is also considering certain insecticides and food additives.

The problems with many of these agents is that it may be some considerable period of time from the exposure to these chemicals before the person develops cancer.

Physical agents

The physical agents which act as human carcinogens are ionizing and ultraviolet radiations. Prolonged exposure to intense sunlight over many years carries an increased risk of cancers of the exposed skin, particularly in fair-skinned caucasian people. In addition, repeated exposure to radiation increases a person's risk of developing cancers. This was first found with the high incidence of skin cancer in people who were making X-ray tubes, and in radiologists, who were unaware of the dangers to which they were exposed.

Viruses

Viruses have been implicated in the causation of cancers in animal experimentation. It is suspected that viruses may play a part in lymphomas, leukaemias and breast cancer. Research continues in this area and has been the subject of further interest with the occurrence of certain rare cancers, e.g. Kaposki's sarcoma, in people who have the human immune deficiency virus which has then led to acquired immune deficiency syndrome.

These groups of intrinsic and extrinsic causative factors play a part in the chain of events leading to a person developing a form of cancer. There is also the view that how the person feels about themselves and the way they generally lead their lives is involved in the development of cancer (see page 175).

PREVENTION AND EARLY DETECTION OF CANCERS

Although not all cancers can be prevented, people can reduce their risks of developing cancers through avoiding known risks and by their involvement in early detection. If changes are noted when they are still at a precancerous stage, then the chances of a successful outcome to any intervention is much higher.

Nurses have an important role to play in educating people as to risk factors, how to detect for early changes, and in the importance of early intervention. The American Cancer Society has produced a list of early warning signs of cancer:

C—Change in bowel or bladder habit
A—A sore that does not heal
U—Unusual bleeding or discharge
T—Thickening or lump in breast or elsewhere
 I—Indigestion or difficulty in swallowing
O—Obvious change in wart or mole
N—Nagging cough or hoarseness

This is similar advice to that produced by the Health Education Council and cancer societies in this country:

– Watch for any change in your normal state of health.
– Have a medical and dental examination.
– Find out about any lump or sore that does not heal.

- Have a cervical smear test at least three-yearly (the frequency required for this test is under considerable debate).
- Protect yourself against too much sunlight.
- Do not smoke.
- Examine breasts or testes every month.

The nurse can provide this knowledge in a variety of settings. In hospital they can advise the person and their family on wards, in out-patient departments, in clinics and in accident and emergency departments. In the community there are a variety of nurses who can provide this information, e.g. occupational health nurses, health visitors, school nurses, district nurses, practice nurses and community psychiatric nurses.

As nurses we must not only advise people of what to watch for, and what to avoid, but also how to carry out self-examination and what to do if a person is concerned.

The mass media also have an important role to play in educating people. Documentary programmes, radio phone-in programmes, the inclusion of a 'popular' character on a well-watched/listened to programme carrying out health promotion, and the use of leaflets, posters and magazine articles, are just some of the ways in which the mass media can help.

Government also has a role to play through policy and resource decision making. Fiscal policy through taxation on products known to be harmful, e.g. cigarette smoking, the allocation of resources for screening services, and a commitment to policies where expenditure is being provided in the short term for long-term improvement in health, are some of the ways in which government policy can influence this area of health education.

Nurses have a vital role in providing knowledge and education in their interaction with those they care for, through their workplace, and as informed citizens within a community so as to lessen the risk of those we care for developing cancer. It is only by empowering people through knowledge and understanding that we can assist them in the promotion and maintenance of their health.

CARING FOR A PERSON AND THEIR FAMILY WHO HAS DEVELOPED CANCER

Assessment

The physical problems that a person may develop as a result of cancer will depend on which tissue the cancerous cells involve, the extent of that involvement and whether any spread has occurred.

The psychological problems that may occur for the person and their family depend on their understanding of what cancer is, the type of interpersonal relationships and support that exist within the family, their spiritual beliefs and their view of the interventions that are planned.

Areas to consider during assessment of their feelings are:

- Anxieties and fear of the word cancer. Previous knowledge, experience and understanding may shape these anxieties. They may regard it as a death sentence.
- Fear of loss—feelings of denial, anger, bargaining, depression and acceptance may be present in the person and their family (see page 72).
- Loss of self-esteem and dependence. Feelings that their body may have failed them and changes in feelings of worth may be present.
- Feelings of being out of control or having lost control may be evident.

- Loss of body image and changed feelings over their sexuality may be present.
- Feelings of divine retribution or spiritual disillusionment may be present. Guilt—what have I done to deserve this—why me?
- Anxieties over how partners, children or other members of the family will cope.

These are a range of areas that a nurse should consider during assessment. An individual and their family will naturally all react differently and the key to defining problems and planning care will depend on the skill with which assessment is carried out.

It is important that assessment involves the family. A person cannot be nursed without an understanding of how their family feels. Feelings of guilt, especially if there have been problems in the relationship, may be present. The family may start to distance themselves as part of the bereavement process, or want everything tried, irrespective of the person's own views, or a relationship may be strengthened.

Although many of the physical and psychological problems may be present as a result of a large range of different diseases, an essential difference is the term cancer. It has so many connotations for people that it can alter the framework in which care is given. An understanding of what is meant by the term, and the interventions that are planned, are critical if care is to be given well. To quote the American Cancer Society, the person, the family and nurses should remember that 'cancer is a word, not a sentence'.

Surgery, radiotherapy and chemotherapy

Different cancers are treated by surgery, radiotherapy, chemotherapy, or a combination of these approaches.

Surgery

Surgery plays an important part in the management of people with cancer. Surgical biopsy of tissue, or excision of part or whole of an organ, may be considered. In addition, palliative surgery, to reduce particular problems, may be used. Surgical intervention can be minor, as in the case of removal of basal cells, or major, as in removal of a whole organ and surrounding tissue, with resulting severe changes in body image.

The physical nursing interventions are the same as for any individual who has had that part of their body operated upon. However, the psychological care will need to consider the person's feelings as to whether all the cancer has been removed and any spread has occurred. Surgery may also be the first stage of intervention, with chemotherapy and/or radiotherapy planned.

Radiotherapy

Radiation, which is composed of electromagnetic waves, or streams of nuclear particles from atoms of a radioactive substance, may be used to reduce or remove the presence of cancerous cells. It may be given as external radiation, or from a radioactive source placed within the body.

External radiation: This is normally given by a megavoltage X-ray machine, which gives a sharply defined radiation beam with a minimal side scatter of rays. It is planned so as to allow for penetration to the site of the cancer, with as few changes to the other areas of the body that the rays pass through as possible. The strength of these X-rays, the number of treatments, and a shield to protect other parts of the body, are planned by radiotherapists. This treatment must be given in a shielded room.

Internal radiation: Radioisotopes may be introduced

into the body, or applied topically, to deliver radiation to an area where cancerous cells are present. The radioactive elements that are given may be encased or sealed with a non-radioactive metal and inserted into a body cavity, or may be unsealed and given in liquid form.

Radioisotopes that are sealed may be given via needles, seeds, wires or moulds. They are placed within tissue, or a body cavity, for a prescribed period of time, and then normally removed. Depending on the form of internal radiation, a shielded room and specialized equipment may be required.

Nursing intervention

Problem

Anxieties and fears over radiation.

Actions

- Assess the person's understanding of radiotherapy. Misconceptions of the purpose of radiotherapy may be present.
- Explain the type and method of radiotherapy that is to be used.
  - If external radiotherapy is to be used then explanation will be required of the type of machinery, the reasons for isolation during radiotherapy, length and number of treatments and that the person will feel no pain as a result of radiotherapy. Many people have all or part of their course of radiotherapy while staying at home.
  - If internal radiotherapy is to be used then the isolation and protective precautions should be explained to the person and their family. It is important to stress that any precautions are temporary and are

for the protection of family/friends and for those working in the hospital. The length of time radiotherapy is planned for should be stated.

- Spend time listening and answering any queries or worries that the person and their family may have.

External radiation

Problem

Potential for skin breakdown and/or removal of radiotherapy marking.

Actions

- Assess skin for signs of redness, dryness and signs of damage.
- Assess radiotherapy markings. The radiologist will have outlined the area at which the radiation beam is to be directed. These markings should remain until the treatment is finished.
- Ensure that area is not washed, or creams and lotions applied. The friction involved in washing or applying solutions may not only remove the marking, but also cause damage to the layers of the skin below the surface.
- Do not apply pressure or adhesive tapes to the area.
- Do not expose marked area to direct sunlight.

Problem

Nausea and vomiting.

Actions

- Be aware that nausea and vomiting may occur. This

is dependent on the area of the body undergoing radiation.

- Anti-emetics may be required before radiotherapy and before meals.
- Ensure that there is a receiver within reach of the person.
- Give mouthwashes if vomiting has occurred.

Problem

Weakness, fatigue and the need for rest.

Actions

- Allow periods of rest.
- Maintain an adequate nutrition and fluid intake.
- Explain the importance of food and fluids. Good nutrition is important to assist the body with healing as it replaces the lost tissue destroyed by radiation.

Internal radiation

Problem

Need for precautions during internal radiation.

Actions

Assess need and type of precautions required in order to protect other people. Areas to consider are:

- The person may require nursing in a single shielded room.
- Ensure that the person can communicate with nurses on the ward.

- The nurse's time in the room should be restricted to a minimum.
- Ensure that nursing staff are wearing a badge whereby the amount of radiation exposure that they are receiving can be monitored.
- Ensure that the correct disposal of any excreta is understood.
- Ensure that radiation notices are prominently displayed.
- Be aware of the length of time the implant should remain in the body.
- Be aware of the precautions that are required when the treatment is finished.

Problem

Education of the person and their family.

Actions

- Ensure that the person understands about the type of implant they are to receive and any special position that they need to maintain or advice that they must follow.
- Ensure that they understand that they are not a risk to others when the treatment is concluded.
- Ensure that the family understand the restrictions that are required and how they may best communicate with the person undergoing radiotherapy.

In addition, it is important to assess and plan the care required for any of their activities of daily living that they require help with, prior to the beginning of internal radiation. This enables the nurse to ensure that they can plan care in advance, so as to remain in the room for the minimum period of time.

172 MEDICAL NURSING

Chemotherapy

The use of drugs, either on their own or in conjunction with radiotherapy and/or surgery, has become increasingly important in the management of people with cancer. A wide variety of types of drugs are now used, either singly or as a combination of drugs. The commonest groups are: alkylating agents which act within the nucleus of a cell; antimetabolic agents which function at a specific stage of the life-cycle of a cell; plant alkyloids which block cell reproduction; certain antibiotics which inhibit some types of neoplastic cells; and hormones which alter the synthesis of RNA and proteins.

Many of these drugs are highly effective, but may have severe toxic side-effects. A number of these drugs are effective on malignant cells, but may also damage normal tissue. New drugs are being introduced all the time. The common drugs and the combinations in which they are used for different cancers can be found in a specialist textbook.

The drugs used for cancer can be administered in a number of ways: orally, intramuscularly, intravenously, intrathecally, intra-arterially and intracavity. Intravenous drugs may be administered via a central vein for people requiring long-term therapy. In these cases a catheter may be inserted purely for the giving of drugs which is then sealed when not in use. This allows the person receiving those drugs greater mobility.

The drugs which are used are very toxic and specific instructions as to their preparation, administration and side-effects must be carefully followed. The nurse must be aware of the side-effects in order to plan the care and education of the people receiving them. These side-effects can be widespread. They involve, among others, problems resulting from depressing the bone marrow and depressing the immune system, and changes in body image due to factors such as loss of hair.

The nurse must therefore be alert to the range of problems that can occur. Depression of bone marrow may cause weakness and fatigue due to anaemia; a lowered or depressed immune system may cause a drop in the person's white blood count and so make them particularly susceptible to infection—protective isolation may be needed (see page 65). Hair loss may cause anxiety and distress. In addition, some of these drugs interfere with the blood clotting process by causing thrombocytopenia, leading to haemorrhage.

Nursing intervention

Problem

Lack of knowledge of need for education and advice.

Actions

- Assess knowledge and understanding of the person and their family.
- Ensure that they understand the reasons they are on the drug, the dose they require, the length of time each drug is required for and any side-effects that may develop.
- Ensure that they understand the reasons for any restrictions due to the drug therapy such as protective isolation.
- Ensure that they understand the care of any long-term catheter that has been inserted.

Problem

Possible development of side-effects, e.g. potential to develop bleeding or infection.

Actions

- The nurse must ensure that they understand the effects and possible side-effects of the drugs that the person has been prescribed.
- This understanding will allow the nurse to assess for the development of any problems and to plan their care so as to lessen the risk of these side-effects. As an example, if a person has an increased likelihood of developing infection, then the nurse who cares for that person should not have an infection, such as a cold, themselves.

Problem

Potential to develop a sore mouth. Stomatitis (inflammation of the oral mucosa) is not uncommon for people receiving chemotherapy.

Actions

- Ensure good oral hygiene.
- Maintain a moist and clean mucosa.
- Mouthwashes should be given frequently.
- Ensure that dental care is encouraged.
- Antifungal agents such as nystatin may be prescribed to lessen the risk of infection.

Problems

Nausea, vomiting and anorexia.

Actions

- Assess whether anti-emetic drugs help. A wide variety of these drugs are available and are often used for people undergoing chemotherapy.

- Ensure that both the quantities and the types of food are appetising to the person.
- Assess whether the mouth is sore, as this makes eating more difficult.
- Mouthwashes before and after meals may be of help.

Problem

Changes in self-image.

Actions

- Assess likely risk of change in self-image.
- Temporary loss of hair (alopecia) may result.
  Use of wigs, scarves, etc. may help.
  Ensure that the person understands that their hair should grow again.

Despite the problems that can occur, chemotherapy continues to increase in use. It can be responsible for reduction, remission or the removal of cancerous cells. As pharmacological developments continue, this is a form of intervention which is likely to increase.

Complementary approaches to people with cancer

There has been an increasing interest in complementary approaches to caring for people with cancer. This approach is based on the philosophy that cancer is like a seed, but that in order to flourish it must be in the right soil. The person themself is the soil, and therefore that person must make their own environment inimical for the growth of cancer cells. In addition to the concept of the seed and soil, it is often believed that there is some circumstance that sets in train the initial growth of the cancer. This may be a deep emotional stress which must also be dealt with. Cancer can be seen as an opportunity to restructure one's life. Although the cancer may always be with you, you will maintain control over how it expresses itself.

It can be felt that the approach of conventional medicine may deal skilfully with the physical problems of a cancer, but does not adequately help a person to return to normality after having faced a life-threatening experience.

The approach is to treat cancer holistically—the body, the mind and spirit must be looked at together. Cancer cannot be dealt with by simply attacking cancer cells. This perhaps reflects a view, prevalent in other cultures' philosophy of medicine, that where and how a person develops cancer is a reflection of that person's whole being.

The physical aspects of care in relation to basic health of the body involve a change in diet to natural organic foods, fresh vegetables and fruit, and an avoidance of animal protein. In addition the importance of getting plenty of oxygen and exercise is stressed.

The psychological aspects of care are related to learning to relax the body, meditation and visualizing the attack on the cancer in one's body. Counselling for the person and their partner may be offered to help look at the emotional stresses and trauma in life. Relaxation therapy, aroma therapy and the use of touch and massage may also be considered important approaches.

It is argued that this approach can be complementary and not antagonistic to conventional medical approaches. Physicians can excise growths, irradiate and provide chemotherapy. They are concerned with attacking the cancer cells. The holistic complementary approach is to change the environment in which cancer has developed and also to do something about what triggered it off in the first place—to change the circumstances so that a recurrence will be less likely.

Conclusion

The word cancer can be terrifying. It can be associated with death and helplessness. However, nurses can play an important role in allaying these fears. Through our understanding that cancer is a group of problems, we can help a person and their family to see how their own individual health is altered, rather than be submerged by the word they have heard. Through our knowledge of the nature of the problems and the types of intervention that are planned, we can assist the person in understanding their care, and support them during the implementation of that care.

Critically, we have a vital role to play in promoting health and lessening the risk of cancers; by educating people about reducing risk and understanding about the importance of early detection. We can also, in our own lives, act healthily. We can also persuade those we work with and governments to adopt policies designed to promote health and lessen the risks of people developing cancer.

FURTHER READING

DOWNIE, P. A. (1978). *Cancer Rehabilitation. An Introduction for Physiotherapists and the Allied Professions*. Faber and Faber, London.

ERIKSSON J. H. (1989). *Oncology Nursing* (Springhouse notes). Springhouse Publishing Co., London.

FAULDER, C. (1989). *The Womens' Cancer Book*. Virago Press Limited, London.

KAPTCHUK, T. & CROUCHER, M. (1986). *The Healing Arts*. (A Journey Through the Faces of Medicine.) BBC.

LEWITH, G. T. (1985). *Alternative Therapies. A Guide to Complementary Medicine for the Health Professional*. William Heineman Books, Oxford.

MARINO, L. B. (1981). *Cancer Nursing*. C.V. Mosby, St Louis.

TIFFANY, R. (1980). *Oncology for Nurses and Health Care Professionals*, Vol 1. George Allen and Unwin, London.

TIFFANY, R. (1980). *Oncology for Nurses and Health Care Professionals*, Vol 2. Harper and Row, London.

TIFFANY, R. (Ed.) (1981). *Cancer Nursing Update*. Proceedings of the 2nd International Nursing Conference. Baillière Tindall, London.

9 Nutrition

Nutrition is essential for human life. The basic purpose of eating is to provide the nutrients necessary to allow growth of body cells until adult stature is reached and to replenish the substances needed to maintain an adequately functioning body.

Illness has two effects on nutrition. First, the requirements for calories, protein and other essential ingredients may be altered. Second, the ability to consume, digest or utilize these nutrients may be affected.

The role of the nurse is critical in maintaining a patient's nutrition. They are in a position to assess a person's nutritional status, advise on the dietary changes required due to a specific illness, and to help provide nutrition.

This chapter will consider the balanced diet, the assessment of a patient's nutritional needs, and the nurse's role in the provision of oral, enteral and parenteral nutrition. Dietary needs related to specific problems are discussed in the relevant chapters.

THE BALANCED DIET

A normal balanced diet consists of:

Proteins
Carbohydrates
Fats
Mineral salts
Vitamins
Roughage
Water

To function effectively, each cell in the body needs these substances. A balanced diet will contain an appropriate amount of each.

Energy requirements vary widely according to age, sex, occupation and climate. A sedentary man in hospital would need about 10 500 kJ/day, whereas a woman would need 8800 kJ/day. It is important to remember that in many illnesses, energy requirements and protein break-down are increased.

Proteins

Proteins are required for growth, maintenance and repair of body tissue, for the production of enzymes, hormones, antibodies and plasma proteins, and for the production of heat and energy.

A healthy adult requires 70–100 g of protein/day. Proteins are obtained from lean meat, fish, egg whites, cheese, milk, nuts, cereals, peas and beans. Their energy yield is 17 kJ/g.

Carbohydrates

Carbohydrates are required for the production of heat and energy, for the oxidation of fats, for the formation of adipose tissue, to spare protein being used for energy production, and to provide roughage.

A healthy adult requires 400–500 g of carbohydrate/ day. Carbohydrates are obtained from cereals, bread, potatoes, root vegetables, cane sugar, jam and fruits. Their energy yield is 17 kJ/g.

Fats

Fats are required for production of heat and energy, for maintenance of cell structure, to transport fat-soluble vitamins, and for the formation of adipose tissue.

A healthy adult requires 80–100 g/day. Fats are obtained from butter, cheese, cream, fat meat, oily fish, nuts, sunflower and corn oil. Their energy yield is 37 kJ/g.

Mineral salts

The most important minerals are potassium, calcium, sodium, phosphorus, iron, magnesium, chlorides and sulphur.

Potassium helps to maintain the osmotic balance between intracellular and extracellular fluid. It is essential for muscle contraction. It is found in fish, meat, vegetables and citrus fruits.

Calcium is required for the growth of bones and teeth, for the clotting of blood, and for normal muscle function. It is found in milk, cheese, flour, bread and vegetables.

Sodium is required for the formation of bone, for osmosis in the extracellular fluids, for electrolyte balance and for the flavouring of food. It is found in fish and meat. It is added to food during cooking and at the table in the form of sodium chloride.

Iron is needed for the formation of haemoglobin. It is found in red meat, liver, egg yolks, wholemeal bread and vegetables.

Phosphorus, magnesium, chlorides and sulphur are present in all foods.

Vitamins

Vitamins A, D, E and K are found in fatty food and are fat-soluble vitamins. The vitamin B eomplex and vitamin C are water soluble.

Vitamin A is needed for growth and for the protection of surface tissue and certain parts of the eye. It is found in animal tissues, especially in liver and liver oils. Vitamin A is added to margarine.

Vitamin D is required for the metabolism of calcium and phosphorus and therefore the growth of bone and teeth. It is found in milk, butter, fats, fish, and fish-liver oils.

The role of vitamin E in the body is unclear. It is present in all foodstuffs.

Vitamin K is essential for the formation of prothrombin in the liver. It is found in many green vegetables.

The vitamin B complex includes vitamins B_1, B_2 and B_{12}. Vitamin B_1 (thiamine) is needed for metabolism of carbohydrates. Vitamin B_2 is needed for cell metabolism. Vitamin B_{12} prevents the development of pernicious anaemia. The vitamin B complex is found in meat, liver, eggs and cereals.

Vitamin C is necessary for the formation of connective tissue and for the integrity of capillary walls. It is found in citrus fruits, root and green vegetables.

Roughage

Roughage forms the bulk of faeces and helps to stimulate peristalsis in the gastrointestinal tract. It is found in vegetables, fruits, cereals, wholemeal bread and bran.

Water

Water is present, in a high proportion, in all plants and animals.

ASSESSMENT OF A PERSON'S NUTRITION

There are a number of factors to be considered when assessing a person's nutrition:

Ability to swallow and absorb food
Dietary restrictions or needs related to the illness

Physical ability to eat and drink independently
Dietary likes and dislikes
State of mouth and teeth
Cultural/religious needs or restrictions
Appetite
Number of meals normally eaten
Quantity of food normally consumed
Age and sex
Height and weight
Home environment

These factors form the basis on which the nutrition of a person can be planned. The dietician will be involved, with the nurse, in assessing the dietary needs of the person.

In planning a person's diet, it is very important to consider their home environment. A diet given in hospital, where it can be controlled, is of limited use unless the person understands their particular needs and is able to continue the diet when at home.

Nutrition can be given in three ways:

orally
enterally (nasogastric feeding)
parenterally (intravenous feeding)

The nurse has an important role in each of these methods of giving nutrition.

ORAL NUTRITION

Many hospitals provide meals on a hotel-style basis. Menus are given out for people to complete and food is placed on individual trays, which are served and cleared away by junior nurses or non-nursing staff. Thus, the role of the nurse has been reduced. This is to the detriment of care, as it prevents the nurse from assessing nutritional intake and from giving advice.

Assessing nutrition at meal times

As nutrients are essential for the repair of body tissue, it is important that nurses know what people under their care have eaten. In addition, they must be aware of changes in peoples' appetites.

Knowledge of nutritional intake and appetite provides information about the health of a person. Poor nutritional intake may indicate a deterioration in a person's condition. Poor appetite may reflect anxiety or depression. This information is necessary to help assess medical care. Without the nurse's involvement, this knowledge is unavailable.

A further reason why nurses must be involved at meal times is that a number of people will have dietary restrictions. They may need advice or education on what they should or should not eat. Therefore nurses must ensure that serving and clearing away food does not become a non-nursing duty.

Nursing intervention

Presentation and serving of food:

- The way food is presented and served is important in making it desirable. If food is neatly arranged on a plate, the person will feel like eating. The principle is the same as in a restaurant, where, if food was piled up and gravy slopped over the edge of the plate, one would not want to eat it.
- Many people like a drink with their meal and this should be provided.
- If trays are used, the cutlery and condiments should be

carefully arranged. Tray cloths make a surprising difference to the amount of food eaten.

- Meals should be served in a calm and unhurried manner. They are not a task to be quickly finished, but a vital part of a person's care.

Nursing actions:

- The nurse ensures that the person is positioned correctly. Sitting up, well supported, in a bed or chair, makes eating easier and lessens indigestion.
- The nurse ensures any aids required are present, e.g. non-stick mats, adapted cutlery, plate guards, etc.
- The nurse ensures that dentures are clean and in the person's mouth.
- Mouth care may be required before and/or after meals.
- If the food presented is not wanted, replace it with other foods or supplements of equal nutritional value.
- Food should be of the same consistency as the person is accustomed to eating at home.
- If the person requires feeding by the nurse, this should be done in an unhurried way with the nurse sitting down. The person should be given time to enjoy the food. It is helpful to offer fluids at regular intervals when feeding someone, as it often helps digestion. It also serves to slow down the meal and thereby counteract a tendency to complete it quickly.

Food supplements

Normal meals may not always provide adequate nutrition. Difficulty with swallowing, general malaise and debilitation, or specific dietary needs, may mean that oral food supplements are needed.

There are a variety of supplements available. Some are complete foods, e.g. Express Dairy feeds or Ensure, while others consist of specific nutrients, e.g. Caloreen or Hycal. With the help of the dietician it is possible to find a particular food supplement that the patient enjoys.

Food supplements are extremely helpful in giving the patient sufficient nutrition. They may be used to eating only one meal daily. This may not provide adequate nutrition for their particular illness or general condition. Supplements may be easier to take than an extra meal.

The early timing of the evening meal in hospital will not suit all individuals, and some may keep food in their locker. It is necessary to be aware of how much and what foods the person is eating in this way; otherwise, the nutritional assessment is inaccurate. In addition, they may be eating food that is inadvisable, for example a person with diabetes may be eating ordinary chocolate.

Advice on discharge

Nutrition may remain as important in maintaining health at home as it was in hospital. Dietary advice should be given on the basis of the person's home, family, economic status, physical capabilities (including their ability to get to the shops and cook for themselves), level of understanding, particular illness and general health.

Advice should be given throughout the person's stay in hospital. They should choose their own food, with nursing supervision, rather than be given the correct diet. This will help them learn which foods they should be eating.

The whole family should be involved, so that they understand the dietary needs required and can offer support and encouragement. This can be particularly helpful when dietary restrictions are difficult for the person to adhere to, for example reducing diets or abstinence from alcohol.

The dietician should be involved in giving advice to both the individual and their family.

The nurse's involvement and role in oral nutrition cannot be overstressed, as poor nutrition may delay recovery.

ENTERAL NUTRITION

Feeding via a nasogastric tube is the appropriate way of providing nutrition in any patient who cannot eat enough for their requirements *yet* have a normally functioning gastrointestinal tract.

People who will need nutritional support by this means are:

People with a low intake, e.g. anorexic or unconscious people

People with disorders of the upper gastrointestinal tract, e.g. carcinoma of the oesophagus

People with high nutritional requirements due to catabolic states such as burns, multiple trauma or sepsis

There are two methods of enteral feeding: bolus feeding and continuous feeding.

Bolus feeding

This is becoming less common. A wide-bore tube is passed via the nose into the stomach. The prescribed feed is given every three hours using a syringe attached to the tube. The stomach contents are aspirated prior to each feed.

Bolus feeding is important when delayed gastric emptying is present. The wide-bore tube allows aspiration to be performed and thereby ensures that the stomach is empty. However, this method is not often used as it is of less nutritional benefit than continuous feeding, the procedure is time consuming, and the size of the tube makes it uncomfortable for the individual concerned.

Continuous feeding

Feeding via a fine-bore nasogastric tube is used more often than bolus feeding. A fine-bore tube is passed via the nose into the stomach. The prescribed feed is delivered continuously using a reservoir and giving set (Figure 9.1). Its rate of delivery is often controlled by a pump. This ensures that the feed is given at a constant rate and thereby aids absorption. These tubes are much more comfortable than wide-bore tubes. A wide variety of tubes, delivery systems and pumps are available.

If the person is being enterally fed because of a low intake or high nutritional needs, they may eat and drink in addition to the enteral feed.

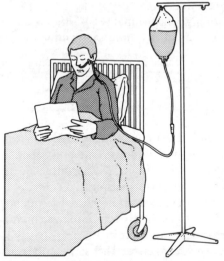

Figure 9.1   Continuous enteral nutrition.

Types of feed

People vary widely in their daily nutritional needs and
no formula is ideal for everyone. Conditions vary from
starvation to the severe catabolism seen in sepsis and
burns. Feeds may be made up by a diet kitchen or may
come direct from the manufacturers. There are a variety
of proprietary feeds available and a knowledge of their
composition is necessary for prescribing enteral feeds. Not
all of these feeds are milk based.

Nursing intervention

Bolus feeding:

- A careful explanation of the procedure should be given
  before the nasogastric tube is inserted.
- The position of the tube is checked by injecting air into
  it with a syringe, while listening with a stethoscope for
  the sound of air entering the stomach, or by aspirating
  some of the gastric contents with a syringe and testing
  their pH. Gastric contents should be acidic, i.e. they
  should have a low pH level.
- Aspiration of the gastric contents should be carried out
  before each feed is given.
- The temperature of the feed should be 37°C when it is
  given. As the feed will have been stored in a refrig-
  erator, it is important to check it has reached the right
  temperature. Water is given after the feed to keep the
  tube patent, and the tube is then closed with a spigot.
  Fluid input and output are recorded.
- The feed must be administered slowly and by gravity. If
  it is given too quickly there is a danger of vomiting and
  aspiration of the feed.
- Drugs may be given at the same time, in liquid or
  powder form.

Continuous feeding:

- Explanation of the procedure is required.
- The position of the tube is checked by injecting air (see above), as it is less easy to aspirate the gastric contents. If any doubt is present, the position of fine-bore tubes can be checked by X-ray as they are radio-opaque.
- Feeds are usually given at half strength for the first 24 to 48 hours to aid absorption. They will then be changed to full strength and the volume increased so as to meet the person's nutritional needs. Fluid input and output are recorded.
- Administration of the feed may be aided by a pump. This controls the flow so that feed is given at a regular rate.
- Fine-bore tubes should be flushed with 5 to 10 ml of water six-hourly to ensure they remain patent. However, with the consistency of modern tubes, fine-bore tubes are unlikely to block up.
- If a person is also taking oral food and fluids, it is helpful to stop feeding via the nasogastric tube an hour before meal times, so as to encourage his appetite.
- People are weighed daily when in hospital.
- Drugs may be given via a three-way tap.

In addition to feeding via a nasogastric tube, food is sometimes given directly into the stomach or jejunum. This is administered via a gastrostomy or jejunostomy tube.

PARENTERAL NUTRITION

Parenteral nutrition is the administration of nutrients directly into the venous circulation. It is used to promote healing and recovery and to replace lost tissue in people when it is *impossible* to provide adequate nutrition via the gastrointestinal tract.

The types of people who are likely to need intravenous feeding are:

Those with gross sepsis causing prolonged paralytic ileus
Those in the pre- and postoperative phases of major
    surgery, especially those with gastrointestinal disease
Those with severe trauma or burns
Those with severe system failure where the gastrointestinal
    tract needs to be rested

Many nutrient solutions are hypertonic and irritant to small peripheral veins. Parenteral nutrition is therefore usually administered into a wide central vein, where rapid dilution with blood reduces the damaging effect. Usually a catheter is inserted via the subclavian vein into the superior vena cava. The end of the catheter will remain on the anterior chest wall 8–10 cm from the clavicle (Figure 9.2). Sometimes the cubital, jugular, cephalic or basilic veins are used.

Electrolytes are assessed daily, and the type of feed prescribed according to the person's particular needs. Drugs may be given with the feed.

Parenteral nutrition is a potentially hazardous therapy, as the person is subjected to risks of:

infection
metabolic disturbance
vascular damage
emotional problems

Infection of the blood by bacteria or fungi is a potential problem because:

Nutrient solutions are an excellent culture medium
An inert catheter is situated in a vein for a long period of
    time
The outside of the catheter provides a possible route of
    direct entry for organisms to the blood.

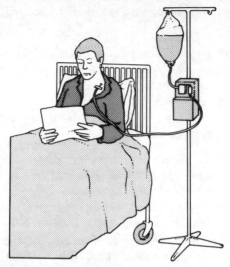

Figure 9.2 Parenteral nutrition.

Metabolic disturbance can occur when large volumes of hypertonic solutions are infused.

Vascular damage may occur due to:

air embolism
catheter blockage
catheter fracture
catheter leakage

Emotional problems may occur; being deprived of oral food and drink for a long period can cause anxiety and distress. The psychological and social needs which are normally met by eating are unfulfilled.

It is the nurse's responsibility to minimize these risks and to ensure that the parenteral nutrition is administered safely.

Problem

Infection control.

Actions

- Asepsis must be carefully maintained during all procedures concerned with parenteral nutrition. Changing the infusion set and performing the dressing to the catheter where it emerges onto the skin are the two main procedures performed.
- The inclusion of all the nutrient solutions needed, including the fat emulsion, in a single container has reduced the risk of infection, because the infusion set needs to be changed only once every 24 hours.
- Individual hospitals have their own procedures for changing infusions.
- The nurse records the person's temperature six-hourly, and observes the skin at the catheter entry site to look for signs of infection.

Problem

Metabolic disturbance.

Actions

- Accurate control of the infusion rate is essential because sudden or slow infusion of nutrients such as glucose or potassium causes severe metabolic disturbance. There are a variety of mechanical devices available, perhaps the most beneficial of which is the volumetric pump.
- Blood glucose levels are measured as hyperglycaemia can occur. In the initial period this may be done six-hourly. Urine may also be assessed for glucose.
- A careful record of fluid input and output is kept. This should be done from parenteral feed to parenteral

feed and not from 12 midnight to 12 midnight. It may be necessary to collect urine or other fluid over 24 hours to estimate nitrogen and electrolyte loss.

- The person is weighed daily. Any signs of oedema are reported.

Problem

Vascular damage.

Actions

- The nurse should take great care with the equipment used.
- Using Luer-lock connections, securing the tubing by adhesive tape, using an extension tube between the catheter and infusion set, and using atraumatic clamps when the intravenous set is disconnected will all help prevent vascular damage.

Problem

Emotional problems.

Actions

- The nurse can help allay some of the feelings of anxiety and distress by having a positive attitude. Parenteral nutrition is not permanent; it is a form of treatment needed only until the main problem is resolved.
- Exercise is important, where practical, for both psychological and physiological reasons. It provides a change of environment and helps assure the person that they are recovering.
- Mouth care helps in both an emotional and physical way. Sucking of boiled sweets can be particularly beneficial.

Parenteral nutrition is life-saving for many people. It is an important method of nutritional support, and its use is increasing. The nurse must remember that, even with good organization, parenteral nutrition remains a potentially hazardous therapy.

ROLE OF THE CLINICAL NURSE SPECIALIST IN NUTRITION

Some hospitals are appointing a clinical nurse specialist concerned with nutrition. These posts may be hospital and community based. The advent of nutritional supplements and enteral and parenteral nutrition means that a nursing source of expertise for people, their families and nursing staff is required.

Advice may be needed on the range of different equipment that is now available. A variety of tubes, reservoirs and pumps are available and the clinical nurse specialist can give advice and ensure consistency of use of equipment within a hospital setting.

They can also help with ensuring that sound nursing guidelines for the use of enteral and parenteral nutrition exist and for the education of nurses in the skilled administration of these forms of nutrition.

These nurses often work as part of a nutritional team consisting of physicians, pharmacists, dieticians and nurses.

They can also help to plan the care and support of people who continue to have enteral or parenteral nutrition in the community. As nutrition may need to be given for a period of time, these methods of nutritional support may be continued outside hospital. This causes a range of problems which community and hospital nursing staff may not feel they have the expertise to manage. Clinical nurse specialists in nutrition have proved invaluable for the support, expertise and skill that they can offer in these situations.

FURTHER READING

BECK, M. E. (1977). *Nutrition and Dietetics for Nurses*. Churchill Livingstone, Edinburgh, London and New York.

BERNARD, M. A., JACOBS, D. O. & ROMBEAU, J. L. (1985). *Nutrition and Metabolic Support of Hospitalized Patients* (Saunders Blue Book Series). W.B. Saunders, London.

BURTIS, G., DAVIS, J. & MARTIN, S. (1988). *Applied Nutrition and Diet Therapy*. W.B. Saunders, Philadelphia.

CHRISTIE, A. B. & CHRISTIE, M. C. (1972). *Food Hygiene and Food Hazards, for Those Who Handle Food*. Faber and Faber, London.

COATES, V. (1985). *Are You Being Served?* (An investigation into the nutritional care given by nurses to acute medical patients, and the influence of ward organizational patterns on that care.) The Royal College of Nursing, London.

GOODE, A. W., HOWARD, J. P. & WOOD, S. (1985). *Clinical Nutrition and Dietics for Nurses*. Hodder and Stoughton, London.

HUSKINSSON, J. (1985). *Applied Nutrition and Dietetics*, 2nd edn. (Current Nursing Practise Series.) Baillière Tindall, London.

QUILLMAN, S. M. (1989). *Nutrition and Diet Therapy*. (Springhouse notes.) Springhouse Publishing Co., Springhouse, Pennsylvania.

10 Nursing people with problems of their gastrointestinal system 1

Disorders of the digestive tract include conditions which affect the alimentary tract (Figure 10.1) from the mouth to the rectum. This chapter will consider the problems people have when their digestive tract is not functioning normally. The problems resulting from abnormal physiology of the related organs—the liver, biliary system and the pancreas—will be considered in the next chapter.

There are a number of areas that a nurse should consider when assessing a person with problems of their gastrointestinal tract. However, these problems are not always caused by a disease process.

Assessment

Dysphagia—difficulty or discomfort in swallowing

Dyspepsia—indigestion

Nausea— the sensation of 'feeling sick', sometimes associated with giddiness and feeling faint

Vomiting—forcible ejection of the contents of the stomach

Haematemisis—vomiting of blood

Melaena—passing of blood into the colon and rectum

Constipation—infrequent and/or difficult passage of faeces

Diarrhoea—frequent passage of loose or fluid faeces

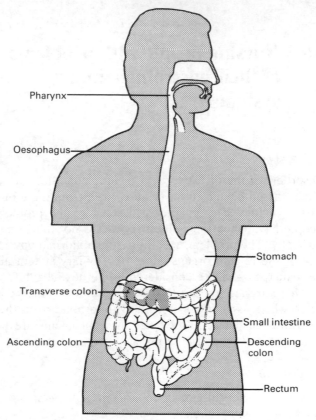

Figure 10.1 The gastrointestinal tract.

Pain—different types of pain can be present. The nature and type of pain, e.g. retrosternal pain (heartburn), abdominal pain or pain on defaecation are important clues as to the particular part of the gastrointestinal tract that is damaged.

Weight loss

Poor appetite
Lethargy and weakness

INVESTIGATIONS

There are two main forms of investigations used on people with problems of the gastrointestinal tract: radiography and endoscopy.

Radiography

A radio-opaque substance (barium sulphate) can be used to outline the gastrointestinal tract. The name of the type of barium X-ray will refer to which part of the gut is being examined.

Barium swallow—oesophagus
Barium meal—stomach
Barium meal and follow through—stomach and small
    bowel
Barium enema—large bowel

Endoscopy

Endoscopes allow visual examination of areas of the gastrointestinal tract. They can also be used to take a biopsy (sample) of tissue. Which investigation is performed will depend on the area to be studied:

Oesophagoscopy—visual examination of the oesophagus
Gastroscopy—visual examination of the stomach
Colonoscopy—visual examination of the colon
Sigmoidoscopy—visual examination of the rectum and
    sigmoid colon

It is also possible to take biopsies of the jejunum using an endoscope.

PROBLEMS OF THE MOUTH AND PHARYNX

Lesions or infections of the oral mucosa can be localized or widespread. If the mucosal involvement is widespread it is termed stomatitis; disease of the tongue is glossitis, of the lips, cheilitis, and of the gums, gingivitis.

Stomatitis

There are several types of stomatitis which vary in form from simple inflammation to vesicle formation and ulceration.

Types

1. Infection with *Candida albicans* (thrush)—a yeast-like fungus.
2. Ulcerative stomatitis—commonly seen in children who are malnourished.
3. Apthous stomatitis—a common cause of stomatitis in infants and young children. It is caused by the virus herpes simplex. Vesicles appear which may rupture and form ulcers.

Some systemic diseases such as syphilis, pernicious anaemia, leukaemia, tuberculosis, smallpox and chicken-pox can cause stomatitis.

Problem

Sore infected mouth.

Actions

- A swab or scraping from a lesion is sent for bacteriological examination.
- Assist with providing appropriate antiseptic lozenge, e.g. domiphen bromide (Bradsol), or antifungal agent,

e.g. nystatin, or antibiotic, e.g. penicillin. The type of drug prescribed will depend on the nature of the organism.

- Mouth care is essential and should be carried out before and after eating.
- Assess how it is most appropriate to provide adequate nutrition and fluids.
- If the organism may cause cross-infection then disposable crockery will be required.

Tonsillitis

Tonsillitis is an acute infection of the tonsils which involves, to varying degrees, the peritonsillar and pharyngeal tissues. The causative organism is usually *Streptococcus haemolyticus*, but a number of other micro-organisms can be responsible. It is primarily a disease of children and young adults.

Problem

Raised temperature (may be as high as 39–49°C) due to infection.

Actions

- Assess temperature.
- Assist with monitoring prescribed antibiotics. These are prescribed, not only to assist the body's defences against the infection, but also to lessen the likelihood of peritonsillar abscess (quinsy), renal damage and rheumatic fever.
- Other measures to reduce the high temperature may be required (see Chapter 3).

Problem

Pain and soreness on swallowing.

Actions

- Aspirin gargles before meals, or antiseptic lozenges, may be given.
- Mouth care is required every two hours.
- Food may be more easily swallowed if soft and a high fluid intake is necessary.

As recurrent attacks of tonsillitis can cause partial obstruction of the nasopharynx, partial deafness due to blockage of the pharyngotympanic (eustachian) tubes, and frequent absences from school, surgery is often considered. A tonsillectomy and removal of adenoidal tissue may be performed when the person has recovered from the acute infection.

Ulceration of the pharynx

Pharyngeal ulcers have a number of causes. These can range from tuberculosis or syphilitic infection, malignant growths (in particular, carcinoma of the tonsillar area) or a type of sore throat known as Vincent's angina. The care required will depend on the primary cause of the ulceration.

PROBLEMS OF THE OESOPHAGUS

The oesophagus is a tubular organ with a fairly simple anatomical structure and a straightforward function. Despite this, it may give rise to a complex set of problems.

Hiatus hernia

A hiatus hernia occurs when a portion of the stomach moves up into the chest through the oesophageal hiatus (opening) of the diaphragm. The hernia may not be present all the time. It may occur only on lying down or when the intra-abdominal pressure rises on coughing or straining.

Hiatus hernias are usually classified into two types: (a) sliding and (b) rolling or paraoesophageal.

Assessment

- Epigastric discomfort
- Dyspnoea
- Palpitations
- Cough

(N.B. these four problems occur due to the slowness of the hernial sac to empty after meals, causing mediastinal pressure.)

- Pain and nausea:
  - on beginning meals (heartburn)
  - after lying flat
  - sometimes on going to bed or changing position
  - on bending down for long periods—e.g. after gardening
  - may extend down one or both arms and simulate angina
- Dysphasia and vomiting due to oesophagitis
- Weakness due to haematemisis and anaemia
  - iron deficiency anaemia with blood in the faeces
  - haemorrhage with haematemisis
  - associated peptic ulceration

An oesophagoscopy, barium swallow or meal and a chest X-ray may be necessary to confirm that a hiatus hernia is present.

Care is concerned with advice as to reducing the severity of the problems. This is normally sufficient, but occasionally surgery is required.

Advice

- Small bland meals should be taken and the evening meal should be eaten at least three to four hours before retiring.
- Antacids, e.g. aluminium hydroxide, are taken after meals and before going to bed.
- The head of the bed should be raised by about 23 cm to help prevent reflux into the oesophagus. If this is not practical then pillows may be placed under the top of the mattress.
- Activities involving bending or stooping should be restricted. Long-handled equipment in the home or garden should also be used to lessen the amount of bending that the person is required to do.
- Weight and diet are assessed. Obesity is fairly common in people who have hiatus hernias. Their problems will be lessened if weight reduction occurs. Advice from a dietician may be helpful.

Gastro-oesophageal reflux and oesophagitis

Although reflux of acidic gastric contents occurs in most people from time to time, it usually passes unnoticed. If reflux becomes frequent, problems may develop. Inflammation of the oesophagus—oesophagitis—may occur due to reflux of either gastric or duodenal contents. Gastric juice contains acid and the enzyme pepsin, both of which can damage the oesophageal mucosa. Duodenal contents, which contain bile and pancreatic enzymes, may reflux through the pylorus into the stomach, and in turn into the oesophagus, causing oesophagitis.

Assessment

Pain (heartburn)
– a burning sensation in the stomach and oesophagus

- mainly retrosternal
- may radiate to back, neck, jaw and arms
- may occur after a large meal
- exacerbated by weight gain
- precipitated by change in position, e.g. lying flat or bending down

Nausea and vomiting due to reflux of acid

Pneumonia may occur in severe cases due to aspiration

Advice

The advice required to lessen the effect of these problems is the same as that given to people with a hiatus hernia (see previous section).

Carcinoma of the oesophagus

Carcinoma of the oesophagus is primarily a disease of elderly people. Lymph node involvement occurs relatively early and there may be a downward spread that can involve the liver. An oesophagoscopy with biopsies and a barium swallow will be carried out to establish whether cancer is the cause of the person's problems. Although the prognosis for a person with this problem is poor, much can be done to alleviate the distress and suffering which is caused, particularly by the accompanying dysphagia.

Assessment

- Dysphagia—onset is often gradual and steadily increases in severity
  (Difficulty in swallowing occurs when about half the circumference of the oesophagus is involved and may be associated with poor co-ordination of the oesophageal contractions. At first the person will have difficulty swallowing solid food such as meat, but as the

dysphagia increases they may become unable to swallow their own saliva.

- Weight loss due to inadequate nutrition. This is more noticeable if there is liver involvement.
- Pain is not normally present unless the cancer is wide-spread. Despite the lack of pain, thirst and excessive salivation make this problem very distressing for the individual.

Medical treatment

Medical intervention for carcinoma of the oesophagus may be by either surgery or radiotherapy. However, as this problem is normally seen in elderly people, and may have been progressing for some time, they are often too ill or frail to undergo major surgery. Consequently, radio-therapy may be chosen. This is aimed at relieving prob-lems and not curing the cancer.

Some form of intubation of the oesophagus may be considered to relieve the dysphagia. This will enable the person to have adequate nutrition and fluids and so maintain the quality of life. Types of prosthetic tubes that are used include the Souttars tube, the Mousseau-Barbin tube and the Celestin tube.

Gastrostomy tubes have been used to ensure adequate nutrition, but should only be used if it is thought that the person's general health will be improved to such an extent that surgery will be possible.

Nursing intervention is aimed at providing emo-tional and psychological support for the person and their family and ensuring that adequate nutrition and fluids are maintained.

Achalasia

The inability of the lower oesophageal sphincter to relax after swallowing is known as achalasia. Oesophageal motility is abnormal. As sphincter relaxation is incomplete, the normal passage of food to the stomach is obstructed.

Assessment

- Dysphagia—intermittent at first
- Regurgitation
  - common
  - food/fluids do not tast sour or bitter, unlike refluxed bile
  - worse on lying down, especially at night
- Pneumonia and lung abscesses may occur if the achalasia is untreated due to aspiration
- Weight loss may occur if the person is reluctant to eat
- Chest pain is unusual

Medical treatment

The intervention for this problem is controversial. The choice lies between dilation and surgery. The majority of people in the United Kingdom are treated by surgical cardiomyotomy—sometimes referred to as Heller–Ramstedt's operation.

Oesophageal varices

The portal venous system communicates with the systemic venous system in the lower third of the oesophagus; here branches of the left gastric vein (portal venous system) and the oesophageal veins (systemic venous system) meet.

If the pressure in the portal venous system rises, it is transmitted from the gastric veins to the veins of the lower oesophagus and varices (dilated veins) can occur. This can happen to people with structural changes of their liver due to cirrhosis or carcinoma (see next chapter).

Oesophageal stricture

Chronic persistent gastro-oesophageal reflux may result in a benign oesophageal stricture. Once an established fibrous stricture has occurred it requires either surgical or endoscopic dilation. Oesophageal dilation is often performed by an endoscopic approach with the person under light sedation (see Figure 10.2).

People may required dilation at three- to six-monthly intervals. Following this procedure people should be assessed for the possibility of perforation.

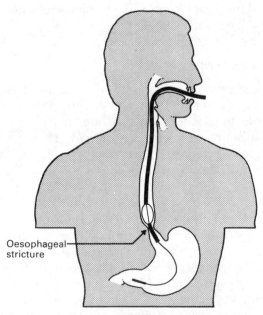

Oesophageal stricture

Figure 10.2 Dilation of an oesophageal stricture using an Eder–Puestow dilator.

PROBLEMS OF THE STOMACH

Peptic ulcers

It is common practice to describe both gastric and duodenal ulcers as peptic ulcers. A peptic ulcer is the erosion of a circumscribed area of tissue in the wall of the gastrointestinal tract that is accessible to gastric secretions. The actual erosion is caused by the digestive actions of hydrochloric acid and pepsin. The ulcer penetrates the mucosa and may invade the underlying submucosal and muscular tissue.

There is no conclusive understanding of the reasons why peptic ulcers form. Normally hydrochloric acid and pepsin are secreted but no ulceration occurs. This is because several defensive factors in the body exist to prevent damage being done to the stomach and duodenum. It is thought that a peptic ulcer develops due to two physiological changes, or a combination of these factors:

1. The secretions of hydrochloric acid and pepsin are in excess of normal.
2. The protective mechanisms in the stomach and duodenum are inadequate in relation to the amount of acid and pepsin that is produced.

Some of the factors that make it more likely that a person will develop a peptic ulcer are:

- Stress. Emotional tension, anxiety, frustration and stress may cause an imbalance in the autonomic nervous system, resulting in an increased vagal stimulation of gastric secretion.
- Heredity. Genetic factors appear to have a role as there is a tendency for ulcers to develop more commonly within families and people of a certain blood group.

There is a correlation between duodenal ulcers and blood group O and gastric ulcers and blood group A.

- Trauma and serious illness. A person with severe tissue damage such as that produced by severe burns may develop peptic ulcers.
- Gender. Peptic ulceration has a much higher incidence in men than in women. It has been suggested that oestrogen hormones in the female may account for this.
- Certain drugs. Some drugs, such as acetylsalicyclic acid (aspirin) and indomethacin (Indocid), are likely to predispose a person to develop an ulcer.
- Diet. Poor dietary habits with irregular meals and long periods between meals may cause hypersecretion of acid.
- Smoking. A high percentage of cigarette smoke is absorbed into the stomach and may cause irritation and damage to the mucosal lining as well as increasing acid secretion.

Other factors which have been sited include: alcohol, bile reflux, excess gastrin concentration in the blood, social class and geographical location.

Admission to hospital is not always necessary. It may be that the person's home situation and their understanding and acceptance of the care and advice they require mean that they can progress satisfactorily at home.

Assessment

- Epigastric pain
  - usually central
  - may vary from over the sternum to over the umbilicus
  - ranges from minimal discomfort to severe
  - usually associated with meals
  - may come on one to two hours after meals

- may wake the person in the early morning
- may be relieved by food, alkalis and vomiting
- may come in waves of attacks and last days or weeks
- Vomiting and nausea—haematemisis and/or melaena can occur
- Malaise and weakness due to poor nutrition and possible anaemia
- Anorexia due to pain after eating which means that nutritional intake may have been poor

If these problems persist and the ulcer becomes intractable, or if there has been severe haemorrhaging, or if the ulcer has resulted in some obstruction in the gastric outlet, then surgical intervention may be considered necessary.

Advice/Health education

The nurse has an important role as a health educator so as to relieve the problems that a person suffers from, to aid the healing of the ulcer and to prevent complications and a recurrence of the ulcer. There are four main areas of education that the nurse should consider: diet, drugs, smoking and lifestyle.

Diet

A regular well-balanced diet free of foods which are upsetting to the individual is advised. Foods that people may find difficult to tolerate are coffee, tea, alcohol, highly seasoned foods and foods that form gas.

Drugs

People will need advice on the drugs that they are prescribed and the drugs that they should avoid. There are four groups of drugs that a person may be given:

1. Antacids. An antacid is given to raise the pH of gastric contents. To be effective they must be taken frequently through the day and when the person is awake at nights. They should also be taken an hour after meals as they buffer or lower the effect of the acid secretions in the stomach and duodenum.
2. H_2 receptor antagonists. In the lining of the stomach we have cells which are stimulated by histamine to produce acid. Drugs can be given (H_2 receptor antagonists) which block histamine stimulating these cells. The two commonest are cimetidine and ranitidine.
3. Anticholinergic drugs may be prescribed. They depress gastric secretions and motility. However, because of the possible side-effects of these drugs they are less widely used.
4. Sedatives and tranquillizers. Tension and emotional stress may cause increased gastric secretions and so sedatives can be used for a short period of time.

In addition, people may need advice to avoid drugs which make an ulcer less likely to heal. Examples of these are drugs which contain salicylate, indomethacin and phenylbutazone.

Smoking

People should be advised to stop smoking as the cigarette smoke absorbed into the stomach increases the secretion of acid secretions and so delays the healing of an ulcer.

Lifestyle

People and their families may need advice as to modifying their lifestyle so as to reduce stress and tension. Help with methods of relaxation and rest should be considered.

Carcinoma of the stomach

Carcinoma of the stomach is a common malignant growth. Men are affected twice as often as women; this sex ratio is fairly constant throughout the world, although the incidence of this form of cancer varies considerably from one country to another.

Gastric carcinoma is often discovered late and the tumour has often invaded related structures, including the lower oesophagus pancreas and peritoneum. Lymphatic spread is common. Secondary spread via the bloodstream leads to involvement of the liver, lungs, brain and bone.

Assessment

- There are often no particular problems at first, although some anorexia and weight loss may be noticed by a person.
- As the tumour develops the person may feel:
  - dysphagia
  - fullness after eating
  - severe epigastric pain
  - weak, lethargic and tired

Surgical resection of the tumour is considered. However, results may be poor due to the difficulty of detecting this form of cancer early enough and secondary involvement may have occurred by the time it is diagnosed.

DISORDERS OF THE SMALL AND LARGE INTESTINE

Ulcerative colitis and Crohn's disease

These are both chronic inflammatory diseases of the gastrointestinal tract. In both cases the cause is unknown.

Although these diseases can affect all age groups, they commonly begin in late puberty and early adulthood. The incidence of both diseases is increasing and both are more likely to occur in women than in men.

In both Crohn's disease and ulcerative colitis there is a known association with other diseases.

In ulcerative colitis:

- Carcinoma of the colon—especially if ulcerative colitis is longstanding and poorly controlled.
- Skin involvement—leg ulcers and skin rashes may be present. Erythema nodosum—bright tender nodes on or below the knees or on the forearms—can occur.
- Arthritis—usually of knees and ankles.
- Eye lesions—iritis.
- Liver disease—cirrhosis of the liver, hepatitis and sclerosing cholangitis may be present.

N.B. The inflammation of the skin, joints and eyes disappears when the inflammation of the colon is under control.

In Crohn's disease:

- Arthritis—often of knees.
- Skin rashes—eczema is common.
- Uteric obstruction and hydronephrosis.
- Problems may arise due to internal fistulae.

In aiding the diagnosis of these problems people may undergo barium X-rays, or endoscopy, and will require stool cultures to be sent for culture and sensitivity, ova and parasites and amoeba. These latter problems can cause severe inflammation of the rectum and colon in their own right.

Assessment

- Pattern of defaecation

Table 10.1 Differences between ulcerative colitis and Crohn's disease.

Ulcerative colitis	Crohn's disease
1. *Areas of the gastrointestinal tract involved*	
Involves the rectum and large bowel	May involve the whole of the gastrointestinal tract. However, about 50% of people with Crohn's disease only have problems in the colon and terminal ileum
2. *Distribution/spread of inflammation*	
Continuous spread of inflammation. This begins in the rectum and spreads up along the colon	Patches of inflammation occur
3. *The layers of the gastrointestinal tract involved*	
The mucosa and submucosa are involved	All three layers of the gastrointestinal tract may be involved
4. *Presence of fistulae*	
Fistulae are not present	Fistulae can occur. These can be either external or internal fistulae. When a fistula occurs it forms a sinus which can track up to emerge on the surface of the skin (external fistula) or the sinus can track into another organ (internal fistula), e.g. a recto-vaginal or oesophageal-tracheal fistula could occur
5. *The size or width of the gastrointestinal tract*	
Normal—although an enlarged colon (toxic megacolon) can occur	The patches of inflamed bowel can narrow down to form strictures
6. *Abscess/ulceration of the gastrointestinal tract*	
Deep ulceration of mucosa and submucosa	Patches of ulceration occur. Abscesses of mouth and anus are common

- How many times a day does the person normally open their bowels?
- How many times a day are they now opening their bowels? This can vary from two to 30 times a day.
- Have they got urgency of defaecation? This can be a crippling problem.
- What sort of faeces are they passing? Assess for presence of:
  - consistency
  - blood
  - mucus
  - undigested food
  - steatorrhoea
- Level, type and areas of pain
  - Abdominal, crampy pain may be present as the bowel may go into spasm.
  - They may have pain or soreness of defaecation.
  - What helps with the pain?
  - How long does the pain last?
- Assess mood
  - Problems may occur in late puberty/early adulthood and people can feel very low, depressed and withdrawn.
- Assess nutrition
  - Have they lost weight?
  - What foods agree and disagree with the individual?
  - Are they taking any nutritional supplements?
- Assess skin
  - Skin rashes, leg ulcers or erythema nodusum may be present.
- Assess eyes
  - The person may have sore eyes due to iritis.
- Assess general physical health
  - The person may be shocked due to pain, frequency of defaecation and dehydration.

- The person may have a fever due to infection.
- They may be weak and lethargic.
- Their skin may be dry and inelastic due to dehydration.

People can present very differently. They may have an acute flare-up and be critically ill or may have been admitted to hospital for rest and alteration of their medication.

Problem

Diarrhoea, frequency and urgency of defaecation.

Actions

- Assess the person's normal pattern of defaecation.
- Ensure easy access to a lavatory. It may be necessary to have a commode by the bed. A side room may be considered.
- Observe faeces and record on a stool chart. Note consistency, frequency, amount of blood, presence of mucus and undigested food.
- Provide handwashing facilities and assist the person to maintain their dignity.

Problem

The person may feel unclean and undignified.

Actions

- Do not communicate any feelings of disgust verbally or non-verbally.
- Privacy for defaecation.
- Ensure that the person has use of air sprays or deodorants to use after defaecation.
- Allow the person to wear their own clothes.

Problem

Pain.

Actions

- Assess level, type and duration of pain.
- Assess whether position helps. People may be helped by lying down on their side with their knees drawn up.
- Assess use of heat pads.
- Assess use of emollient cream or local anaesthetic gel for use after defaecation.
- Assess effectiveness of drugs. Analgesia does not often help as the pain is due to spasm. Antispasmodic drugs may be more beneficial.

Problem

May have low mood and depressed range of feelings.

Actions

- Assess mood and feelings.
- Show empathy. Demonstrate that you are aware of how miserable it must be to have this range of problems.
- Ensure that the person understands that you do not think they are a difficult or demanding person. Their problems occur as a result of their ill-health and not because they are an 'awkward' person. There is no evidence that personality plays any role in causing ulcerative colitis or Crohn's disease. As a result of the frequency of bowel actions and the age at which these complaints normally occur, it is perhaps not surprising that people can become somewhat withdrawn and anxious.
- Attention to appearance may help. Wearing of own clothes may increase self-esteem.

Problem

Dehydration and malnourishment.

Actions

- Assess nutrition and fluid intake. People may be able to eat normally or may require nothing to eat and drink in order to rest their gut.
- Ensure that nutritional needs are met by the provision of food and fluids that the person can absorb. People vary widely as to which foods they can tolerate. This must be assessed individually.
- Involve the dietician for advice.
- Present food attractively.

Problem

Weakness, malaise and lethargy.

Actions

- Assess whether bed-rest is required.
- If bed-rest is not indicated, ensure easy access to the lavatory.
- Assess which activities of daily living the person may need assistance with, e.g. hygiene and dressing.
- Allow time to rest without interruption.

Problem

May have poor physical health.

Actions

- Assess the person's physical health.
- Check blood pressure and cardiac rate for shock.
- Assess temperature for infection.

- Assess skin for potential pressure sores, rashes and leg ulcers.
- Assess urine for glycosuria as the person may be prescribed high-dose corticosteroids.

Problem

Need for advice on education on discharge from hospital.

Actions

Assess knowledge and plan a programme of teaching. Areas to be considered include:

diet—how to maintain a balanced diet
drugs—possible need for steroid card and blood count
involve the family in educational programme
follow up medical supervision
employment/financial worries
information on national organization: National Association for Colitis and Crohn's disease, 98a London Road, St Albans, Herts, AL1 1NX.
information on any local support groups

Crohn's disease and ulcerative colitis tend to flare up from time to time. However, as people get older these attacks occur less frequently. In severe cases surgery will be considered. This may involve creating an ileostomy for a person with ulcerative colitis or partial resections of areas of the gastrointestinal tract for people with Crohn's disease. This may be considered when strictures and/or fistulae are present.

An important part of caring for people with these problems is the use of drugs. The nurse should be aware of these drugs, their actions, routes of administration and side-effects. A person may be on medication of various sorts for a considerable period of time and so will need to be knowledgeable and educated about the drugs that they are required to take.

Drug treatment

1. *Drugs used to reduce inflammation.*
   - Corticosteroids—usually prednisolone is used. This can be given orally, intravenously or rectally by suppository or enema. The importance of not stopping these drugs, carrying a steroid card and the side-effects of these drugs must be stressed.
   - Sulphasalazine. This is a non-steroidal anti-inflammatory drug which is particularly effective if inflammation of the colon is present. It may be given orally but can be given rectally by suppository and enema. It can cause skin psoriasis.
   - Immunosuppressive drugs such as azathioprine can also be used. These drugs may suppress a person's bone marrow and they will need to have their blood platelets checked once- to four-weekly.
2. *Drugs to reduce infection.* Antibiotics such as metronidazole or a form of penicillin may be used. These can be prescribed for long periods, e.g. three to six months. As this is unusual the person must be aware that this is what was intended.
3. *Drugs to help with pain control.* Antispasmodic drugs may be given. Buscopan is the commonest, although it is usually given intramuscularly and so is impractical when the person leaves hospital.
4. *Drugs to control bowel frequency and diarrhoea.* A variety of drugs may be given, such as Isogel, codeine phosphate or Lomotil. It is important to remember, that in ulcerative colitis, although rare, severe constipation can occur and so laxatives may be required.
5. *Drugs to help with nutritional support.* It may be necessary to take iron tablets or vitamin supplements. If the terminal ileum is involved, as it often is with Crohn's disease, then replacement vitamin B_{12} by injection may be required.

Diverticular disease

A diverticulum is a herniation of the mucosa through the muscle wall. Diverticula may occur anywhere in the gastrointestinal tract, but they are most commonly found in the colon. When diverticula become inflamed, because of faecal impaction and infection, the condition is known as diverticulitis.

The problems that result from the formation of diverticula vary considerably; people are often problem-free until a complication such as infection occurs. However, if a pharyngeal or oesophageal diverticulum occurs, its presence may cause severe mechanical problems.

Colonic diverticulitis is usually treated by advice on the prevention of constipation—either by dietary changes or the provision of a laxative. In severe cases, hospital admission and possibly surgery may be required.

Carcinoma of the colon and rectum

Carcinoma may occur anywhere in the large bowel but is most commonly found in the rectum and sigmoid colon.

Assessment

The problems will vary slightly according to the site of the tumour.

Pain
- usually not severe
- a persistent, dull ache
- sometimes associated with meals } especially in carcinoma of the
- patient may be afraid to eat } caecum

Alteration of bowel habit
- occurs most often in carcinoma of the descending colon or rectum

– alternating constipation and diarrhoea may occur
Blood and mucus in faeces
– usually means the carcinoma is low in the colon
Steady weight loss

Medical investigation and treatment

- A barium enema followed by a sigmoidoscopy or colonoscopy with biopsies will usually confirm the diagnosis.
- Unless secondary spread has occurred, surgery will normally be performed.

Parasites

There are a wide variety of parasites which may inhabit the gastrointestinal tract. They are commonest where personal or community hygiene is poor, and in tropical or subtropical countries. A wide range of abdominal problems may result with general manifestations of ill health and malnutrition.

Some of the commoner parasites are:

tapeworm
threadworm
hookworm
Salmonella
Schistosoma (Bilharzia)
roundworm
whipworm

Detailed information can be found in specialist textbooks.

FURTHER READING

See Chapter 16.

11 Nursing people with problems of their gastrointestinal system 2

This chapter will consider the problems that a person has as a result of disorders of their liver, gallbladder and pancreas. The anatomical arrangement of these organs is shown in Figure 11.1.

JAUNDICE

Jaundice is a term used to describe the yellow discoloration of the skin which occurs when the serum bilirubin rises above 50 mmol/l. Bilirubin undergoes a series of changes from the time it is produced in the spleen until the time it is excreted from the body. It is formed from haem following the breakdown of red blood cells in the spleen. It is insoluble in water and needs to be conjugated by the liver so that it can be excreted either in the faeces as stercobilinogen or in the urine as urobilinogen (Figure 11.2).

This pathway can be disrupted at different parts of the sequence. Table 11.1 shows the classification of jaundice, which depends on the part of the pathway affected.

As there are a variety of factors that can cause jaundice, it is important that an accurate history is taken from the patient concerning the sequence of his problems.

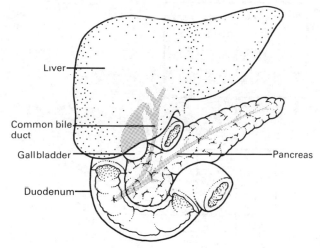

Figure 11.1   The liver, gallbladder and pancreas.

Table 11.1 Classification of jaundice

Failure to conjugate bilirubin
newborn (due to immaturity of the enzyme which conjugates bilirubin)
haemolytic disease
certain drugs
viral hepatitis (occasionally)
Gilbert's syndrome

Failure to excrete conjugated bilirubin
Intrahepatic
   viral hepatitis
   cirrhosis of the liver
   ulcerative colitis
   pregnancy
   carcinoma (primary or secondary)
Extrahepatic (obstructive)
   gallstones in the common bile duct
   carcinoma of the head of the pancreas
   sclerosing cholangitis

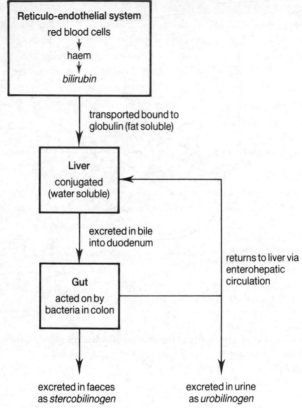

Figure 11.2 The bilirubin pathway.

DISORDERS OF THE LIVER

Liver biopsy

A liver biopsy is often used as an aid to diagnosis in suspected chronic disease of the liver. It is taken by puncturing the liver with a special needle inserted in the mid- or anterior axillary line between the eighth and ninth, or the ninth and tenth ribs. The person's blood group, platelet count and prothrombin time ratio (blood clotting time) will have been assessed prior to this investigation. A liver biopsy is not normally performed if the prothrombin time is more than two seconds longer than the control. If the prothrombin time is raised, vitamin K may be given intramuscularly.

Nursing intervention

- A full explanation of the procedure and of the need for supine bed-rest is given to help alleviate the person's anxiety. A doctor will obtain the person's consent prior to the procedure.
- The person should be lying supine, with their right side at the edge of the bed and their right arm behind their head so as to provide clear access to the chest wall.
- The person may become shocked due to blood loss as the liver is such a vascular organ.
- The blood pressure is assessed at 15-minute intervals initially to monitor for falling blood pressure and an increasing cardiac rate—hypovolaemic shock. These observations will be lessened in frequency as the risk of haemorrhage lessens.
- The wound site should be checked for signs of bleeding.
- Bed-rest in a supine position is maintained for 12 to 24 hours.
- The nurse should also assess respiratory distress and/or pain as the needle may have damaged another organ.

Problems caused by disorders of the liver

People can suffer from a variety of problems due to dysfunction of their liver. This variety is due to the wide-ranging functions of the liver. This section will review those functions, discuss the problems and actions for people with disorders of their liver and then look specifically at the problems people have who suffer from viral hepatitis.

Functions of the liver

1. To assist with the formation and secretion of bile. All the liver cells continually form a small amount of bile which is secreted into bile canaliculi.
2. Storage of glycogen. Glycogen can be reconverted into glucose whenever the blood sugar is too low. The liver is also capable of converting amino acids and glycerol to glucose (gluconeogenesis) should the need arise.
3. Metabolism of fat. The liver cells desaturate fat. This means that it converts stored fat to a form in which it can be used by the tissues to provide energy. The liver also converts excess carbohydrate and amino acids into fat for storage.
4. Deamination of amino acids. The end products of protein digestion are amino acids which are absorbed into the portal circulation through the villi of the small intestine. Many of the amino acids pass through the liver and are used by the tissues for growth and repair. Any remaining amino acids are oxidized to provide energy, or converted to fat or carbohydrate. Deamination is the removal of the nitrogen portion of the amino acid, which is not required for the formation of new protein. The liver forms ammonia from the unwanted nitrogen portion, which in turn combines with carbon dioxide to form urea.
5. Production of plasma proteins. The liver forms 90–95% of the plasma proteins, albumin, globulin and fibrinogen.

6. Storage of vitamins. The liver stores vitamins A, B_{12}, D, E and K. In addition to storing these vitamins, the liver can also synthesize vitamin A from carotene which is found in food.

7. Storage of iron. The liver stores iron in the form of a protein compound called ferritin. The iron is derived from the haemoglobin of worn-out blood cells which have been destroyed by the spleen and from iron absorbed from the small intestine. This reserve of iron is reused for the formation of haemoglobin.

8. Production of heat. The liver uses a considerable amount of energy and has a high metabolic rate. It is the main heat-producing organ of the body.

9. Production of clotting factors. The liver plays an important role in blood coagulation by forming many of the substances involved in the blood clotting process. These include fibrinogen, prothrombin and factor VII. Vitamin K, which is stored in the liver, is needed for the formation of prothrombin and factors VII, IX and X.

10. Detoxification. The liver is able to destroy or modify toxic substances in the body. Many drugs are chemically reduced to simpler non-toxic compounds for excretion by the body or are totally destroyed. Several hormones, including thyroxine, oestrogen and aldosterone, are either chemically altered or excreted by the liver.

Problems and nursing actions

Problem

Confusion—Coma (encephalopathy). This is thought to occur due to failure of the liver to metabolize and detoxify nitrogenous substances. This problem can occur if a person has cirrhosis of their liver, liver failure generally, primary cancer (hepatoma) and occasionally secondary cancer.

Actions

- Assessment of neurological state. Changes in mental state must be reported. A continuum exists of neurological disturbances from mental slowness to full coma. This continuum is classified into four stages or types:
  Type 1: Inappropriate responses
  Type 2: Drowsy/sleepy, but will wake up and respond normally
  Type 3: Continually drowsy, confused and agitated
  Type 4: Coma
- If confusion develops:
  - protein is restricted in the diet. This can be as low as 20–40 g/day. Although the person's level of protein in the blood may be low, restriction may be required because of the damaged liver's failure to excrete the products of protein breakdown.
  - ensure frequent bowel actions. This is necessary to lessen protein absorption from the gut and enable the undamaged part of the liver to work more effectively. Oral laxatives such as lactulose can be used or enemas may be required. Record bowel actions on a stool chart.
  - no sedatives should be given.
- Nursing actions to maintain the person's safety may be required.

Problem

Ascites. This can occur where there is structural damage to the liver. These changes may happen as a result of cirrhosis or cancer of the liver. The reason is thought to be a combination of two factors: firstly, hepatic tissue damage, obliteration of blood vessels and compression of the fibrous tissue cause an increase in blood pressure within the portal vein, and this means that fluid can escape into the peritoneal cavity; and secondly, due to the failure to produce sufficient serum albumin to maintain the normal colloidal osmotic pressure of blood.

Actions

- The person should be nursed sitting upright. It may also be necessary to nurse the person with the head of the bed elevated. These actions will help to relieve pressure on the respiratory system.
- Girth measurements are performed. The abdomen must be marked clearly on both sides so that the same area is measured at each recording.
- Fluid intake may be restricted.
- Fluid intake and output must be assessed. Diuretic drugs may have been prescribed and so a record of fluid output is important.
- The person is weighed daily.
- Sodium in the diet may be restricted. This can vary from advising the person not to add salt to their diet to a formal restriction of 40 mmoles daily.
- If intravenous infusion of fluid is required then 10% dextrose is often used. This is because both normal and dextrose saline obviously contain sodium.

Occasionally abdominal paracentesis is performed. This is now rare because of the changes that occur in electrolyte and protein loss. It may be done for people with advanced cancer where their ascites is causing respiratory distress. This will help to maximize the comfort of the person through this period of their life.

Problem

Liability to bleed. This occurs with cirrhosis of the liver and cancers due to portal hypertension and the disturbance of the formation and synthesis of clotting factors.

Actions

- Early detection of bleeding. The nurse should note any signs of bruising, epistaxses or the development of haemorrhoids. These are early signs that the venous system is under increasing pressure.
- The veins in the oesophagus may be dilated. This is known as oesophageal varices. The danger is that these may burst and this is a life-threatening experience. The care of a person with oesophageal varices is discussed in the references suggested as part of Further reading.
- Vitamin K and a transfusion of blood platelets may be given.
- Any signs of melaena will be reported.
- Blood pressure will be recorded but changes in blood pressure do not occur quickly unless haemorrhaging is occurring.

Problem

Itching of the skin (pruritis) and yellow skin due to jaundice. Conjugated and unconjugated bilirubin may accumulate because bilirubin uptake and excretion may both be defective. Pruritis is caused by the build-up of salts under the skin.

Actions

- Nursing actions are aimed at relieving discomfort. Clean linen and frequent bathing may help.

Soap should be avoided and water should be warm rather than hot. The heat and alkali in the soap tend to increase the discomfort of pruritis.

Calamine lotion may help—largely as a distraction from the awful feelings of continuous itchiness.

Fingernails should be short, filed and kept clean.

- A low-fat diet can be used to lessen the nausea that may be felt.
- Assess urine for bilirubin and urobilinogen.
- Be aware of how the person may feel, as they look different.

Problem

At risk of developing an infection and may be infectious to others. The person may have viral hepatitis and so be infectious to others. In liver failure generally a person may be more prone to developing infections. The reason for this is not clearly understood. It may be due to their general weakness, combined with the possible use of long-term corticosteroid therapy.

Actions

- Non-infectious liver disease
  Nurse upright and encourage deep breathing exercises so as to prevent chest infections.
  Assess for signs of infections, e.g. purulent sputum, infected urine or a wound that is breaking down.
  Assess temperature for pyrexia.
- Infectious liver disease (see section on Viral hepatitis).

Problem

Anxieties, depression and low mood and feelings of isolation can occur. The changes in lifestyle that may be required, the change in a person's colour, fears over their future and altered body image all contribute to these feelings.

Actions

- Assess the person's mood and feelings.
- Explain nursing actions and share knowledge and feelings with the person and their family.
- If the person requires isolation this is a particularly important aspect of their care (see page 67).

Problem

Hyperglycaemic episodes. This may occur due to the reduction in protein, fat and sodium, so high-carbohydrate diet and high-dextrose solutions may have to be used.

Actions

- Assess blood sugars.
  Glucose in urine is assessed. B.M. stix may be used but consideration is given to whether the person has a problem with the blood clotting mechanism.
- If the sugar levels are high, oral hypoglycaemic medication or insulin may be needed. It may not be practical to reduce the carbohydrate in the diet, as the person would be getting very little nutrition.

It must be remembered that drowsiness could be due to encephalopathy and/or changes in blood sugar levels.

Problems

Weakness, lethargy, anorexia and fatigue. These occur due to the widespread effects of liver disorders on the body.

Actions

- Assess the assistance required with activities of daily living, e.g. hygiene, feeding and mobility.
- Assess the skin for risk of decubitus ulcers.

Problem

Need for advice on future lifestyle.

Actions

Assess the person and their family's knowledge and plan a programme of education. Areas of advice that may be necessary include:

- Dietary advice. Changes in amounts of protein, fat, carbohydrate and salt may have been prescribed. Vitamin supplements may also be required.
- Need to abstain from alcohol. Involvement of support services that are available. If liver damage has occurred, people are advised that they may not take alcohol again.
- Need for convalescence. People may feel very weak and lethargic, particularly after viral hepatitis, and convalescence and rest may be needed. This may have financial/employment consequences.
- Drug therapy. People will need advice on the reasons why they are taking drugs, the dose, times when they should take those drugs and the side-effects of those drugs. They may require corticosteroids and so will need advice on this group of drugs.
- Risk of their blood or faeces being infectious and so a risk to others (see Viral hepatitis).

Viral hepatitis

As more than 25% of the output of the heart passes through the liver it is particularly susceptible to any pathogenic organism that gains access to the general circulation or to the portal venous system.

Inflammation and infection of the liver can occur through viruses. Two categories or types of viral infection are viral hepatitis A and viral hepatitis B. A third type of viral hepatitis has been isolated which is known as non-A non-B viral hepatitis. The term Hepatitis C is now being used for non-A non-B viral hepatitis. This section will concentrate on the problems people have as a result of viral hepatitis A and B.

Although the problems people present with as a result of hepatitis A or B are similar, the transmission of these viruses, their epidemiology and the future for people as a result of these viral infections are very different.

Assessment of people with viral hepatitis A and B

Assessment can be divided into two periods: these are referred to as a pre-icteric phase and an icteric phase.

Pre-icteric phase:

The person feels unwell
Nausea and vomiting may occur
Anorexia
Malaise
Severe headaches
Loss of desire for cigarettes and alcohol
Mild fever
Urticaria
Polyarteritis in up to a quarter of people

This range of problems can occur with general ill-health or flu and so can make it difficult to be aware that a person has developed viral hepatitis.

Table 11.2 A comparison of some of the differences between viral hepatitis A and B

Viral hepatitis A	Viral hepatitis B
Age	
Tends to be of children and young adults	No specific age affected
Transmission	
Normally via faecal–oral route. This is where faeces have entered the water supply or food and then be consumed by a person	Normally through blood transfusions, needles and syringes and blood products. Also through sexual activity where blood may be involved. It may be transmitted from the mother to a fetus during pregnancy
Spread	
Epidemics tend to occur. This may be within a community, a family, a school or prison. If food or water is contaminated with infected faeces then it is likely that more than one person will develop this infection	Normally sporadic spread. Nursing staff and health professionals in contact with blood and blood products are highly at risk
Type of virus	
Caused by small RNA virus	Caused by double-shelled DNA virus
Incubation period	
Short—roughly 14–40 days.	Longer period—roughly 40–180 days. This can mean it is hard to be positive about the source of the infection
Presence of antigens/antibodies in the blood	
Antigens and antibodies are not present in blood	Antigens are present in a person's blood. Most people will also develop antibodies
Recovery patterns	
Most people recover without future problems	There are three patterns of outcomes—See section on hepatitis B

Icteric phase:

Jaundice develops
– appears between two and eight days after the end of the pre-icteric phase
– characterized by pale faeces and dark urine

If a person recovers normally, then, as they gradually feel better, their appetite returns and their fever subsides.

As has been stated, although people may present with the same range of problems, the transmission of these viruses, the care and advice required and the outcomes for the person who has viral hepatitis are different as a result of whether they have the A or B virus.

Viral hepatitis A

The main aims of care are to prevent cross-infection of hepatitis A to others and to provide education and support for the person who has developed this viral infection.

Towards the end of the incubation period, the virus may be found in the faeces in the week preceding the onset of jaundice and for up to a week afterwards. During this period the person is at risk of infecting others. The route of infection is obviously through their faeces. If they require admission to hospital then excretion/secretion isolation will be required (see Chapter 4). However, in many cases people are nursed at home. They and their family need careful advice about handwashing after using the lavatory.

Nurses and medical staff will be concerned to isolate the reason for the infection, as measures can then be taken to prevent infection of other people in the community. This is a notifiable disease.

As the jaundice disappears the person begins to feel

better. Generally hepatitis A is a mild, self-limiting infection. Complete recovery, with the liver function tests returning to normal, usually occurs within three months.

For people travelling to areas where hepatitis A is common, vaccination with normal human immunoglobulin can be given. This passive immunity lasts for four to six months. After natural infection with hepatitis A, immunity is lifelong.

Viral hepatitis B

Hepatitis B is caused by a viral infection passed through blood. The problems that a person develops are similar to those of a person who has hepatitis A but may occur more slowly. The major differences are that there are different outcomes for the person and patterns of recovery.

There are three main patterns of viral hepatitis B.

1. Acute infection with recovery.
2. Chronic persistent hepatitis.
3. Chronic aggressive hepatitis.

Most people, about 95%, who have hepatitis B, have an acute infection and recover normally. In a small number of cases, hepatitis B can lead to fulminant hepatitis. This is where the liver fails rapidly and death occurs.

People are diagnosed as having hepatitis B because of the presence of antigens in their body. Three types of antigens are found:

hepatitis e antigen (HbeAg)
hepatitis surface antigen (HbsAg)
hepatitis core antigen (HbcAg)

The first two antigens are found in the blood and core antigen may be found on examining the cells of the liver under the electron microscope. If a person has hepatitis e antigen in their blood, they have hepatitis B.

The pattern of recovery and the advice people will require depend on whether they develop antibodies to these antigens. These antibodies are known as:

antibodies to hepatitis B surface—(anti-HBs)
antibodies to hepatitis e—(anti-HBe)
antibodies to hepatitis c—(anti-HBc)

People tend to fall into three groups. The first develop antibodies to e antigen and core antigen after roughly 4–12 weeks. Antibodies to surface antigen will also develop but over a longer period of time. The second group of people will develop antibodies, but this will not occur for a number of years. The third group of people will not develop antibodies.

These patterns of when, and if, antibodies develop are important for both the person and those caring for them. When antibodies to e antigen develop, the person is no longer regarded as infectious to others. Therefore, one group are potentially infectious for a relatively short period of time, the second group may be at risk of infecting others for a number of years, and the third group are always at risk of infecting others.

Nursing is directed at ensuring that the person does not infect others. Therefore, we need to know whether they have developed antibodies, in order to give the correct advice. People who are admitted to hospital may require isolation as their blood, and any fluid containing blood, constitute a risk to others. However, whether full isolation nursing is required is assessed individually. Some people may be able to be nursed within the normal ward environment with the appropriate care being taken over their blood and any syringes or needles that are used. All specimens must be labelled with a high-risk label.

Advice for someone when they leave hospital is based on whether they remain infectious to others. If they are then they will need advice on what to do if they cut themselves, or require surgery in the future.

Most people recover well from hepatitis B. People who may always be chronic carriers can also feel well and lead normal lives in the community.

Hepatitis B vaccination

Vaccination against hepatitis B is available. Nursing staff who come into contact with blood, body fluids, needles and sharp instruments should be offered the benefit of vaccination against hepatitis B. Although good infection control techniques remain the first and essential component of the prevention of infection, they cannot guarantee protection from hepatitis B as accidents still occur.

Vaccinations are available from general practitioners and occupational health departments.

Neoplastic conditions of the liver

Primary carcinoma of the liver is rare. It is normally associated with a pre-existing liver disease such as cirrhosis. However, secondary deposits in the liver (metastases) are more common. The ratio of secondary carcinoma of the liver to primary carcinoma is 20:1. Metastases usually spread from a primary carcinoma of the gastrointestinal tract, as the malignant cells are carried to the liver in the portal vein. Primary carcinomas of other organs such as the lung and the bronchus may also cause secondary liver involvement.

Treatment is normally palliative, as the primary carcinoma is usually at an advanced stage when the liver involvement is diagnosed. However, cytotoxic therapy and/or surgical resection is sometimes indicated. Liver transplantation has been achieved and there may be further developments in this field in the future.

DISORDERS OF THE GALLBLADDER AND BILIARY TREE

The common diseases of the gallbladder and extrahepatic ducts are infections (cholecystitis) and stone formation (cholelithiasis). Carcinoma is rare.

Standard radiological techniques in investigation of known or suspected biliary tract disease include cholecystograms, percutaneous transhepatic cholangiography and ultrasonography.

Endoscopic retrograde cholangiopancreatography (ERCP)

Endoscopic retrograde cholangiopancreatography (ERCP) has become more widely used as it enables contrast to be placed in high concentration in the biliary tree and pancreas so that excellent X-rays of the biliary and pancreatic ducts may be obtained.

It is most commonly used in investigating obstructive jaundice, disorders of the pancreas and biliary tract disease, particularly if gallstones are suspected. It is carried out under an intravenous sedative, e.g. diazepam. Certain operative techniques can be performed via the endoscope: incisions may be made electrically to allow gallstones to be passed or removed. This is especially useful in people whose general condition may render them unfit for a laparotomy, such as the elderly.

Nursing intervention

Pre-investigation:

- The person should have nothing orally for eight hours prior to the procedure.
- An intravenous infusion is commenced.
- Blood is cross-matched and the prothrombin time ratio

...y if a sphincterotomy is to be per-

...tion is required; consent is obtained by
the ...

• Post...

...re are monitored to detect

...to detect the presence of
...ay cause pancreatitis.
...tics will be given,
...es daily) and/or
...

...owed anything by mouth
...owing ERCP. If a sphincterotomy
has been performed, the person is not allowed anything
by mouth for 24 hours.

Cholecystitis and cholelithiasis

Cholecystitis (inflammation of the gallbladder) may
present as an acute, a chronic, or a subacute illness. It is
more common in females and its frequency increases with
age. It is usually associated with cholelithiasis (gallstones),
but between 10 and 30% of those with inflammatory
changes have no gallstones. Cholesterol is the major constituent of gallstones, especially in Western countries.
They may be single or multiple and, in addition to
cholesterol, may contain bile pigments, carbonate, iron,
calcium, phosphate and protein. They can occur anywhere
within the biliary system (Figure 11.3).

Causes

The aetiology of gallstones is complex and is almost
certainly multifactorial.

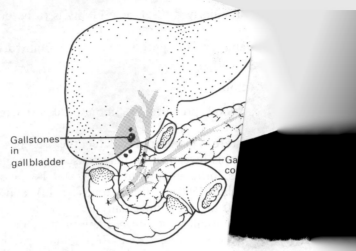

Gallstones
in
gall bladder

Ga
co

Figure 11.3   Gallstones.

Since cholesterol is the major constituent of gallstones, theories usually centre on cholesterol precipitation. However, there is considerable debate as to the nature of this relationship. Diet is also held to be important, and research on the effects of different types of carbohydrate is being done. Stasis, infection and alteration in the composition of bile are a further three factors thought to be relevant to the formation of gallstones. However, there is, as yet, no definitive explanation of the formation and presence of gallstones.

Assessment

Acute severe pain
- deeply seated in the epigastrium
- radiates to the right hypochondrium along the phrenic nerve
- usually comes on suddenly

– may reach great intensity

Nausea and vomiting—may be bile stained

Shock

– pallor

– tachycardia

– low blood pressure

– the person may feel cold and have clammy hands

Fever—may be 38–39°C

Jaundice—if bile ducts are obstructed by a stone or inflammation

Tenderness and guarding of the muscles, especially over the gallbladder

Problem

Pain.

Actions

- Assess pain for type, intensity and duration.
- Analgesia is given to help relieve pain, e.g. pethidine.
- If spasm is occurring, relief can be given by the use of an anticholinergic drug such as propantheline. This lessens the spasm of the sphincter of Oddi (the valve controlling the flow of bile into the duodenum) and so decreases the pressure in the bile ducts.
- Explanation will help to relieve anxiety and in turn the pain felt.
- Assess whether heat pads, touch or massage help.

Problems

Shock and dehydration.

Actions

- Assess blood pressure and cardiac rate.

- Report any changes.
- An intravenous infusion may be required.
- Assess and record fluid intake and output.

Problem

Nausea and vomiting.

Actions

- Assess whether the person should have nothing to eat and drink.
- If this is the case a nasogastric tube may be inserted and nausea and vomiting relieved by aspirating the tube hourly.
- Anti-emetics can be given.
- Mouth care will be required to ease the discomfort of a dry mouth and the taste caused by vomiting.

Problem

Fever.

Actions

- Assess and record temperature.
- Monitor the effects of the antibiotics that may be prescribed. These are normally given intravenously at first.
- If profuse sweating occurs then wash and dry the person thoroughly and help to change their nightwear.

Problem

Anxiety and distress.

Actions

- Explanation and assurance are important as the intense pain can cause fear and anxiety.

- Give clear instructions as to the reasons for nursing actions.
- Allow time for the person to express their feelings.
- Touch and listening may help relieve anxiety.

As the pain and fever subside then fluid and foods are introduced. Food should be low in its fat content. A small amount of fat is helpful as it causes the gallbladder to contract and so prevents stasis of bile.

Health education/advice

Dietary advice will be required as to the amount of fat that it is considered wise for the person to eat. If the person is overweight then restriction of carbohydrate may be necessary. It may be helpful to involve a dietician.

A period of convalescence and rest may also be advised. Assess whether this is practical and whether there are any financial problems. Advice from the social worker may be sought.

Advice on future management will be required. The importance of a follow-up appointment should be stressed. This is particularly important as future surgery and/or an ERCP and sphincterotomy may be planned. Normally surgery or endoscopic intervention is carried out when the problems have subsided and the person has had a period of rest at home. In critical cases, where problems persist, an operation may be required urgently.

DISORDERS OF THE PANCREAS

The problems that people suffer as a result of inflammation of their pancreas or a tumour are considered in this chapter. The problems resulting from diabetes mellitus will be considered in Chapter 14.

Investigation of pancreatic disorders may include ERCP (see page 242).

Pancreatitis

Pancreatitis can take the form of an acute or chronic disease.

Causes

The cause of pancreatitis is not clearly understood and many views have been put forward. It is almost certainly multifactorial. Some factors which are thought to be important are:

Obstruction of the pancreatic ducts
Reflux from the duodenum
Infection, usually secondary; the disease develops in
    association with a focus of infection elsewhere in the
    body, e.g. viral hepatitis
Metabolic factors—hyperlipidaemia occurs frequently;
    also an unexplained relationship between hyper-
    parathyroidism and pancreatitis
Vascular disorders—venous obstruction or reduced ar-
    terial supply
Alcohol

Investigations

Pancreatic function tests. Serum amylase and lipase are monitored as they reveal the degree of duct obstruction and the excretory ability of the pancreas. Pancreatic function is also assessed by taking specimens of duodenal aspirate and blood samples before and after giving injections of secretin and pancreozymin.

Radiology. An ERCP will be performed if the facilities

are available. A plain X-ray of the abdomen may show pancreatic calcification.

On recovery, a cholecystogram and a barium meal are performed to look for gallbladder disease and duodenal ulcer, respectively.

Acute pancreatitis

In acute pancreatitis the changes in the pancreas vary from slight oedema to almost complete destruction by haemorrhage. Infection is not common; if it does occur it is normally secondary. Damage to the pancreas results in the escape of its enzymes both locally and into the circulation, and it is this which is reponsible for most of the person's problems.

Assessment

Epigastric pain
– usually sudden in onset
– severe and continuous
– may radiate through to the back (possibly due to the escape of blood and enzymes into the retroperitoneal space)
Shock
– rapid pulse with poor volume
– pallor
– cyanosis
– low blood pressure
Vomiting
– frequent small amounts of bile-stained fluid
– vomiting of intestinal contents occurs if peritonitis and ileus develop
Rigidity of abdominal muscles
– present, but not marked
– some upper abdominal tenderness and guarding

Fever
– if the inflammation of the pancreas is severe

Problem

Pain caused by inflammation of the pancreas.

Actions

- Assess type, severity and duration of pain.
- Analgesia is given for pain. It is normally felt to be excruciating. Pethidine is often used as it, unlike morphine, does not cause spasm of the sphincter of Oddi.
- Bed-rest is required.
- Assess whether heat, cold, massage or other nursing actions help to relieve pain.
- Anticholinergic drugs such as probantheline may be given to diminish the vagus-stimulated secretion by the pancreas. They also lessen spasm of the sphincter of Oddi.

Problem

Nausea and vomiting.

Actions

- The person is not allowed to eat and drink, so as to lessen the work of the pancreas and allow healing.
- A nasogastric tube is passed which should be aspirated hourly.
- Record all vomiting on a fluid output chart.
- Anti-emetics may help.
- Mouthwashes are required to relieve the person's dry mouth and uncomfortable taste after vomiting.

Problems

Dehydration and shock.

Actions

- Assess blood pressure and pulse.
- Observe for pallor and cyanosis.
- Monitor intravenous infusion.
- Record fluid balance.
- Note urinary output carefully as anuria can develop in severe cases of shock.

Problems

Potential for unstable blood sugar levels.

Actions

- The level of sugar in the blood must be monitored as pancreatic damage can cause high blood sugar levels. If blood sugar levels are high then insulin or hypoglycaemic oral drugs may be required.
- Report if the blood sugar level is outside the normal range.
- Monitor urine for glucose.

The person and their family will naturally be anxious, as the intense pain that is felt causes distress. Other problems that the nurse should be aware of are fever and the possible development of jaundice. In addition, the nurse should assess bowel actions for steatorrhoea—an abnormally high fat content within faeces. This can occur due to pancreatic damage.

Health education/advice

The nurse's role in health education concerns advice about diet and alcohol consumption. If pancreatic damage has resulted in poor blood sugar control, then advice on the amount of carbohydrate that the person should consume is required. In severe cases they may require insulin or hypoglycaemic drugs for a period on leaving hospital.

Alcohol is forbidden. If alcohol intake has contributed to a person's pancreatitis, it may be difficult for them not to take alcohol again and advice and support will be necessary. Family involvement and the support offered by outside agencies are essential.

Chronic pancreatitis

Chronic pancreatitis is characterized by progressive fibrosis and atrophy of the pancreas. It may occur insidiously without pain until the person presents with obstructive jaundice, steatorrhoea or diabetes. Obstructive jaundice occurs due to the infiltration of the head of the pancreas with fibrous tissue. Although pain may not be present, if it is, as with acute pancreatitis, it is severe and intense.

Carcinoma of the pancreas

Carcinoma is found in three areas of the pancreas:

in the ampulla
in the head of the pancreas
in the body and tail

Carcinoma of the pancreas is rare. It accounts for about 1% of all carcinomas. Men are more commonly affected than women. Most occur in those aged 50 to 70 years of age, although other age groups may be affected.

Assessment

Weight loss
Pain

Indigestion

Melaena

Chronic diarrhoea—steatorrhoea may be present

Mild diabetes

Venous thrombosis

Fever

Jaundice

Metastatic spread to the coeliac plexus of nerves may occur

The location and spread of carcinoma in this part of the body, together with the effects on the person, mean that care is normally aimed at maintaining the person's dignity and quality of life.

Surgery offers the main prospect of a permanent cure. However, this is extremely difficult and in itself carries a high mortality rate.

FURTHER READING

BOUCHIER, I. A. D. (1977). *Gastroenterology*, 2nd edn. Baillière Tindall, London.

BRUNT, P. W., LOSOWSKY, M. S. & READ, A. E. (1988). *Gastroenterology*. Heinemann Medical Books, London.

GRIBBLE, H. E. (1977). *Gastroenterological Nursing*. Baillière Tindall, London.

HAMILTON H. & ROSE M. B. (eds) (1985). *Gastrointestinal Disorders*. Nurses Clinical Library, Springhouse Publishing Company, London.

JONES, F. A., GUMMER, J. W. P. & LENNARD JONES, J. E. (1968). *Clinical Gastroenterology*, 2nd edn. Blackwell Scientific Publications, Oxford.

POUNDER, R. (ed). (1986). *Doctor there is Something Wrong with My Guts*. Grangewood Press, London.

RAVENSCROFT, M. M. & Swan, C. H. J. (1984). *Gastrointestinal Endoscopy and Related Procedures*. Chapman and Hall, London.

RYALL, R. J. (1984). *The Digestive System*, 2nd edn. Churchill Livingstone, London.

SHERLOCK, S. & SUMMERFIELD, J. A. (1979). *A Colour Atlas of Liver Disease*. Wolfe Medical Publications, Holland.

SHERLOCK, S. (1985). *Diseases of the Liver and Biliary System*, 7th edn.

Blackwell Scientific Publications, London.
SYKES, M. (ed). (1981). *Aspects of Gastroenterology for Nurses*. Pitman
    Books, London.
THOMPSON, R. (1985). *Lecture Notes on the Liver*. Blackwell Scientific
    Publications, Oxford.

12 Nursing people with problems of their renal system

The urinary system (Figure 12.1) is concerned with:

Excretion of the end-products of protein metabolism
Regulation of electrolyte and water content
Regulation of acid–base balance
Excretion of drugs and poisons
Regulation of blood pressure
Formation of red blood cells
Metabolism of vitamin D
Production of erythropietin for the formation of red blood
    cells

The functional unit of the kidney is the nephron (Figure 12.2). The glomerulus filters blood so that water, electrolytes, glucose, amino acids and waste products flow down the nephron. In the tubule most of the water is reabsorbed together with the glucose, amino acids and some salts. Antidiuretic hormone regulates the reabsorption of water.

Approximately 1.5 l of urine passes out of the tubules each day. This is conveyed from the pelvis of the kidney down the ureters to the bladder and urethra.

The following terms are used to describe abnormal function of the urinary tract:

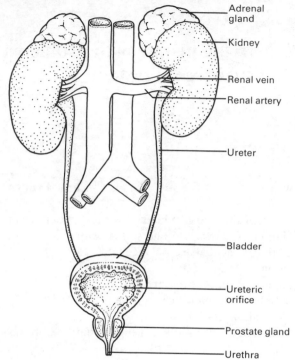

Figure 12.1 The male urinary tract.

Retention—inability to pass urine from the bladder
Retention with overflow—urine is voided but there is a
   residue of urine left in the bladder
Anuria—failure of the kidneys to produced urine
Oliguria—reduction in the amount of urine produced
Polyuria—increase in the amount of urine produced
Haematuria—presence of blood in the urine
Glycosuria—presence of glucose in the urine
Proteinuria—presence of protein in the ruine

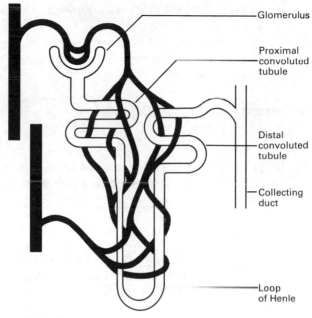

Figure 12.2 The nephron.

INVESTIGATIONS

Examination of the urine

1. *Volume*. Normal range is 600 to 2000 ml per day.
2. *Specific gravity*. Normal range is 1003 to 1030. A low specific gravity indicates concentrated urine.
3. *pH*. Urine is usually acid pH 4 to 6, but becomes alkaline if left to stand. Urinary pH can be measured using a Multistix.
4. *Colour*. Dilute urine is a pale, straw colour. Concentrated urine is a darker yellow. Red or smoky-coloured

urine may contain blood. Yellowish-brown urine may contain bile.

5. *Abnormal constituents*. Blood, glucose, ketones, protein, bilirubin and urobilinogen can be detected by testing with a Multistix.

Bacteriological examination of the urine

A mid-stream specimen of urine should be obtained for microscopy and culture.

To detect the presence of tuberculosis of the urinary tract, all of the first urine specimen of the morning needs to be sent to the laboratory. This is known as an EMU.

Blood urea and electrolytes

These tests are used to detect impaired renal function. Impaired excretion of urine due to diseased kidneys will cause the blood urea and potassium to rise.

Creatinine clearance

The function of the kidneys can be measured by the clearance of creatinine. Creatinine is an end-product of muscle function. It is filtered off in the glomeruli. Calculation of the serum creatinine, the urinary creatinine and the urine volume in a 24-hour period can be used to measure the glomerular filtration rate.

X-rays of the urinary tract

A plain X-ray of the abdomen will show the outlines of the kidneys and the presence of any stones in the urinary tract. Small kidneys may indicate chronic renal failure.

An intravenous urogram (pyelogram) involves an intravenous injection of a contrast medium which is subsequently excreted by the kidneys and therefore outlines the pelvis and calyces of the kidney, the ureters and the bladder. It will reveal any abnormality in shape or size and any obstruction or deformity. A laxative is normally given the day before the examination in order to prevent the urinary tract being obscured by a constipated, gas-filled bowel. Better pictures are obtained if the urine is concentrated and the person should be deprived of fluid before the test (this is contraindicated in renal failure and myeloma).

A retrograde pyelogram involves an injection of contrast medium into the kidneys via ureteric catheters inserted through a cystoscope. The dye outlines the pelvis and calyces of the kidney and the ureter.

A renal arteriogram involves an injection of contrast medium into the aorta close to the renal arteries. To do this a catheter is passed up into the aorta through a femoral artery in the groin. The renal blood supply can then be outlined. This investigation is often performed under general anaesthesia. Vital signs and pedal pulses are recorded because of the risk of haemorrhage from the arterial puncture site. The person should rest in bed for 8 to 24 hours.

Isotope scanning of the kidney

A radioactive isotope is injected intravenously. This is taken up by the tubules of the kidney and a sensor device enables a picture of the isotope concentration in the kidney to be built up.

Ultrasound

Ultrasound of the kidney can detect structural abnormalities such as polycystic kidneys (see page 284).

Renal biopsy

A renal biopsy involves the obtaining of a minute cylinder of kidney tissue for histological examination. This is usually performed using a needle. It is a potentially dangerous procedure with a high risk of haemorrhage. A clotting screen is done prior to the biopsy to ensure that this is within normal range, and blood will be cross-matched in case haemorrhage does occur.

The procedure should be explained carefully to the person, who will then be asked to sign a consent form. It is performed under local anaesthesia. The person should rest in bed for 24 hours after the procedure. Observations are initially made every 15 minutes. All urine is observed for blood.

CYSTITIS

Cystitis is an attack or chronic inflammation of the bladder. It has a higher incidence in females due to the short urethra. The organism commonly involved is *E. coli*, which usually enters the bladder through the urethra.

Predisposing causes

Trauma to the urethra, e.g. mechanical effects of intercourse.
Stasis of urine—incomplete emptying of the bladder.
Distortion or compression of the bladder by enlarged neighbouring organ—e.g. pregnancy.
Poor personal hygiene when toileting.

Assessment

Frequency, urgency, burning pain on passing urine—dysuria

Nocturia—having to get up in the night to pass urine

Suprapubic discomfort

Urine has a strong abnormal smell and is cloudy in appearance

Problems

- Urinary frequency and dysuria related to the presence of the urinary infection.
- Potential for recurrence of infection.

Actions

- Mid-stream specimen of urine is obtained for bacterial examination. (The urine specimen must be collected before any drug treatment is started.)
- Trimethoprim is the most commonly used antibacterial drug used for *E. coli* infection.
- Encourage the person to drink at least three litres/day unless contraindicated. Increased fluids will dilute the urine, which lessens irritation and burning and provides a continual flow of urine to discourage stasis and multiplication of the infecting organism. The problems will usually disappear within 48 hours of commencement of antibiotic therapy.

Education/Support

- Encourage the person to have follow-up urine studies.
- For people with repeated urinary tract infections, encourage good personal hygiene and efficient cleaning of the perineum.
- Avoid external irritants, e.g. bubble baths.
- Certain women are prone to cystitis after sexual intercourse. They should be advised to pass urine before and immediately after intercourse.

- Both partners should be advised to wash themselves before and after sexual intercourse.

ACUTE PYELONEPHRITIS

Pyelonephritis is an acute bacterial infection of the renal pelvis and kidney tissue. It is caused by organisms which have invaded the lower urinary tract and ascended to the kidney via the ureters. Normally the glomeruli of the kidney not only filter the blood passing through them but also destroy the bacteria being carried by the blood. When something happens to interfere with this progress the bacteria may enter and infect the kidney.

E. coli is the organism most commonly involved. Other organisms which may cause acute pyelonephritis include *Klebsiella*, *Proteus*, *Enterobacter* and *Pseudomonas*. Pyelonephritis is far more common in women than in men; this is due to the shorter urethra in women.

Problems

Onset is usually sudden with loin pain and tenderness
Fever 39–40°C.
Rigors
Nausea and vomiting
Malaise
Frequent and painful micturation (dysuria)
Urine is cloudy and may contain bacteria, pus, blood and
    epithelial cells

Actions

- Collect mid-stream specimen for culture of micro-organisms and sensitivity to antibiotics. (Antibiotic therapy is usually then prescribed.)
- Assist in carrying out diagnostic intravenous pyelogram

which will assist in determining the level of the functioning of the kidneys.

- Encourage the person to drink three litres/day unless there is complete obstruction of urinary drainage, or decreased renal function. The recording of the fluid intake and output is necessary in order to detect a reduction in urine output.
- If renal function is decreased, fluid overload could occur, so observe for:
  confusion
  shortness of breath
  peripheral oedema
  sudden weight gain (by assessing daily weight)
- Take temperature six-hourly.
- Fan or tepid sponge the person if temperature rises above 39°C.
- Pulse, respirations and blood pressure are recorded six-hourly.
- A rise in blood pressure may indicate deteriorating renal function.

In recurrent acute pyelonephritis a daily dose of antibiotics may be given long term. Renal X-rays, renal CT scan and an ultrasound would be performed in order to detect any abnormality of the renal tract such as renal stones.

In the absence of any abnormality, recurrent acute pyelonephritis rarely results in chronic renal failure.

Education/Support

Advise the person that a daily dose of antibiotics will need to be taken long term, that a daily increased fluid intake must be maintained, and that urine cultures and evaluation studies will be continued until there is no evidence of inflammation.

ACUTE GLOMERULONEPHRITIS

Glomerulonephritis is an inflammatory non-bacterial disease of the glomeruli. There are three types:

minimal change
proliferative change
membranous

In each of these types, protein leaks through the glomeruli and appears in the urine.

Glomerulonephritis is caused by immunological or allergic reactions affecting the glomeruli. A common antigen causing acute proliferative glomerulonephritis is the bacterium β-haemolytic streptococcus. This organism causes a throat or skin infection and 10–14 days later an allergic inflammation occurs in the kidneys. However, in many cases the antigen causing glomerulonephritis is unknown.

Assessment

Fatigue
Hypertension (with mild, moderate, severe headache)
Fever
Oedema
– generalized
– most noticeable in the face
– due to salt and water retention
Dyspnoea—due to pulmonary oedema
Oliguria
Haematuria
Proteinurea
Uraemia—raised blood urea and creatinine

Problem

Fatigue due to disease.

Action

Encourage person to rest in bed in the acute phase.

Problem

Hypertension—the person may complain of headaches.

Actions

- Monitor six-hourly recordings of blood pressure.
- Offer medication as prescribed to relieve headaches.

Problem

Fluids are restricted to 500 ml each day plus the previous day's output.

Actions

- Measure and record intake and output.
- Offer mouth care two-hourly because of the restricted oral intake.
- Weigh the person daily in order to detect fluid gain or loss.
- Diuretic drugs may be required.
- A 24-hour urine collection may be necessary to estimate the creatine clearance.

Problems

Restriction in dietary protein.
Sodium and potassium intake may also be limited.
Person complains of anorexia.

Actions

- High-carbohydrate diet to provide energy.

- Explain to the person the reason for the fluid and dietary restrictions.
- Daily urinalysis to detect the amount of protein being lost in the urine.

Problem

Risk of deterioration of condition.

Action

- Temperature, pulse and respirations are recorded six-hourly. (If any throat or skin infection is present, swabs will be taken and an antibiotic prescribed, e.g. penicillin may be prescribed by the doctor.)
- Blood will be taken for urea and electrolytes.

Problem

Restriction in activities of daily living due to bed-rest.

Action

For care see Chapter 3.

After a period of two to three weeks, the urinary output increases, proteinurea decreases, and the blood pressure returns to normal. During this diuretic phase the fluid intake is increased to prevent the person becoming dehydrated. Dietary restrictions are lifted and salt supplements may be given.

Education/Support

- The person must understand that if they develop any infection it must be treated promptly.
- They must understand how important it is to have follow-up evaluations of blood pressure, urinary pro-

tein, and blood urea nitrogen level to determine if there is recurrence of disease activity.

• They must recognize if the problems of renal failure are occurring and know to call the doctor immediately.

Conclusion

The majority of children who suffer from acute glomerulonephritis will recover completely. In adults the disease will often progress, eventually leading to chronic and end-stage renal failure.

NEPHROTIC SYNDROME

This is not a disease, but a collection of problems. It is characterized by oedema, proteinuria, and a low serum albumin.

Predisposing causes

Glomerulonephritis
Amyloidosis
Diabetic nephropathy

The excessive loss of protein in the urine results in a low serum albumin. This in turn causes a low osmotic pressure in the blood and consequently generalized oedema results.

Medical investigations

• Nephrotic syndrome caused by glomerulonephritis can be treated with steroids, e.g. prednisolone. If the symptoms fail to resolve, cyclophosphamide, an immunosuppressive and cytotoxic drug, may be used.
• Diuretic and antihypertensive drugs may be given.

Problem

Oedema because of salt and water retention with:

– puffy eyes in the morning
– swollen feet and ankles later in the day
– swollen genitalia

Actions

- Weigh person daily to detect fluid gain or loss.
- Fluid intake and output recorded on chart.
- Blood pressure should be recorded with the person lying and standing as postural hypotension may sometimes occur. The person may find anti-embolic stockings helpful.

Problem

Susceptibility to infection.

Action

Temperature recorded six-hourly.

Problem

Proteinuria (loss of protein in the urine).

– large amount usually found on Multistix testing
– dark foamy urine

Actions

- Urine tested daily for blood and protein.
- 24-hour urine collection to estimate the amount of protein lost in the urine.

Problem

Because of loss of protein in the urine and presence of oedema there will be dietary restrictions.

Action

A high-protein, low-salt diet is given. A low-fat diet may be prescribed if there is hyperlipidaemia (an excess of fats or lipids in the blood).

Problem

Restriction in activities of daily living due to bed-rest necessitated by the condition.

Action

See Chapter 3.

Education/Support

The course of the disease is variable. The person often has multiple hospital admissions and is very conscious of their oedematous appearance. They will need continuing support and explanation. Many people will develop chronic/end-stage renal failure, except for those suffering from minimal change glomerulonephritis.

ACUTE RENAL FAILURE

Renal failure is the inability of the kidneys to function. The substances normally eliminated in the urine accumulate in the body fluids as a result of impaired renal secretion and lead to a disruption of homeostatic, endocrine and metabolic functions. This can cause uraemia, and then renal failure. The person in renal failure cannot independently sustain life.

Predisposing causes

Reduction in renal blood flow
Blood loss (surgery, trauma)
Plasma loss (burns, surgery, acute pancreatitis)
Sodium and water loss (prolonged diarrhoea or vomiting, gastrointestinal drainage and sustained high fever)
Severe infections/Septic shock
Cardiac failure
Crush injury
Poisons
Chemicals
Drugs
Incompatible blood transfusions
Renal causes
Acute glomerulonephritis
Fulminating pyelonephritis
Obstruction to outflow of urine
Prostatic hypertrophy
Renal stones
Tumours

Assessment

Oliguria—urine volume less than 400 ml/24 hours
Anuria—not passing any urine
Effects of decreased urinary output are retention of certain biochemical substances in the blood, e.g. urea, creatine
Potassium and sodium chloride concentrations will cause sodium and water retention, leading to oedema. Unless this is controlled it will lead to cardiac failure
The inability to regulate the electrolytes and excretion of metabolic wastes will lead to:
- nausea
- vomiting

- drowsiness
- confusion
- cardiac arrhythmias
- rapid breathing (Kussmauls)
- gastrointestinal bleeding
- twitching
- coma

Problem

Alteration in elimination of urine due to impaired renal function.

Actions

- Fluid intake will be restricted to 500 ml each day plus previous day's output. A record of the fluid intake and output must be charted to determine the daily volume of fluid to be given. Frequent blood tests of electrolytes are followed closely because sodium and potassium levels are especially important in determining the type of fluid to be administered.
- Weigh the person daily; this will also determine the daily volume to be given (if not ventilated or in intensive care).
- Any oedema is noted.
- Urine is tested daily for blood and protein.

Problem

Potential for cardiac problems due to inability of the kidneys to excrete potassium.

Action

- Pulse, respirations and blood pressure recordings are made frequently. Continuous ECG monitoring may be established if potassium levels remain elevated.

- A rise in blood pressure may indicate fluid overload.
- Temperature is taken four-hourly; a sudden elevation may indicate infection.

Problem

Potential for difficulty in breathing—pulmonary oedema which can result from overhydration and cardiac failure.

Action

- Four-hourly respiratory recordings. An increase in volume and depth of respiration may point to acidosis (an increase in hydrogen content of the blood).
- If the person is short of breath they should be assisted to sit upright and the medical staff informed. Oxygen is given as prescribed.
- In more severe pulmonary oedema, it is helpful if the person sits in a high-backed chair with their legs down. This allows excess fluid to pool in their legs rather than in their lungs.
- Put sputum container and tissues within reach of the person; sputum in pulmonary oedema will be frothy and possibly blood-stained.
- Seek medical advice if problems persist. Venipuncture or haemodialysis may be necessary.

Problem

Alteration in neurological status.

Action

- Assess level of consciousness and orientation.
- Assess muscular twitching.
- This must be noted as it may indicate cerebral oedema and approaching convulsions and coma.

Problem

Alterations in nutritional status due to inability of the kidneys to excrete catabolic wastes.

Actions

- Protein intake is restricted to 20–60 g/day, depending on the severity of the renal failure.
- Offer high-carbohyrate feeding, since carbohydrates have a greater protein-sparing power.
- Glucose solutions such as Hycal and Caloreen may be used.
- Restrict foods and fluids containing potassium and phosphorus, e.g. banana, citrus fruits/juice, coffee.
- Reduce sodium intake as directed.
- Anti-emetic drugs, e.g. metoclopramide, may be required before meals to prevent nausea and vomiting.
- Kaolin mixture, diphenoxylate (Lomotil) or Loperamide are used to relieve diarrhoea.
- Haemodialysis may be necessary to remove the electrolytes, urea and waste products that the kidney is unable to excrete.

If sodium and potassium levels are high, an ion exchange resin (calcium resonium) may be given orally or rectally to reduce the potassium level. If calcium resonium is ineffective, glucose and insulin may be given intravenously to promote the transfer of potassium into the cells, thus lowering the serum potassium. An infusion of sodium bicarbonate may also be helpful.

Problem

Restriction in activities of daily living.

Actions

- Activity is not restricted but most of the individuals

concerned are extremely ill and need help with every activity. (Some people may be nursed in the intensive care unit.)

- People with acute renal failure are lethargic due to uraemia and anaemia. Meticulous skin care is essential to prevent skin breakdown.
- Pruritis may be a problem—chlorpheniramine may be prescribed.
- Position changed frequently and pressure areas protected.
- Strict attention is given to personal hygiene as these people are susceptible to many infections.
- Provide fluid in small amounts; ginger ale and other effervescent soft drinks are tolerated better than other fluids.
- Meticulous mouth care is essential to protect teeth and mucous membranes.

The diuretic phase of acute renal failure occurs 10–21 days after the onset. Increasing amounts of urine are passed; this is very dilute at first. Renal function gradually improves, although it may be several months before it returns to normal. During the diuretic phase, fluid and electrolyte balance must be watched carefully. Fluid intake is calculated.

Sodium and potassium supplements may be required and the dietary restrictions may be lifted. Urine collections for creatine clearance will be performed in order to reassess renal function.

Education/Support

The person and family must understand that activity should be resumed gradually and that they will need to continue with plenty of rest. The person must understand the importance of avoiding any infection.

Dietary instructions may need to be given to the person and family by the dietician. An appointment will be made for the person to see the social worker if socio-economic support may be required.

The person will be closely supervised by the medical staff as an out-patient until fully fit and healthy.

The person may have chronic renal failure in the future if the impairment of the kidneys is permanent, but usually recovers fully.

CHRONIC RENAL FAILURE

Chronic renal failure is irreversible impairment of renal function.

Predisposing causes

The main causes of chronic renal failure are:

chronic glomerulonephritis
pyelonephritis
polycystic kidneys (see page 284)
malignant hypertension
diabetes

Other less common causes include analgesic misuse, tuberculosis and amyloidosis.

Glomerulonephritis often accompanies collagen diseases such as systemic lupus erythematosus (SLE), polyarteritis nodosa (PAN) and scleroderma.

Assessment

Chronic renal failure will cause disturbance of most systems of the body. Therefore assessment will be required of:

Skin
- pallor due to anaemia
- scratch marks due to pruritis
- bruising due to platelet deficiency

Gastrointestinal
- nausea and vomiting
- diarrhoea
- anorexia
- thirst
- hiccoughs
- dry, coated tongue

Cardiovascular and respiratory
- hypertension
- chest pain
- oedema
- dyspnoea
- frothy sputum
- hyperventilation

Blood
- anaemia
- lethargy
- bleeding tendency

Urinary
- oliguria, anuria
- proteinuria
- haematuria

Neurological
- insomnia
- lack of concentration
- drowsiness
- confusion
- coma
- fits and twitching
- numbness in legs

Muscular
- cramps
- weakness

Bone
- pain
- osteomalacia

Eyes
- deteriorating vision

Endocrine
- impotence
- menstrual disturbances

Medical treatment

The management of chronic renal failure includes dietary restrictions, fluid and electrolyte restriction and sometimes medication. End-stage renal failure is treated with dialysis and transplantation. Dietary, fluid and electrolyte control are discussed on pages 271–3.

People with end-stage renal failure who cannot be treated with dialysis or transplantation will require terminal care.

In the early stages of chronic renal failure most people have polyuria and therefore the fluid intake should be liberal. In the later stages the urine output decreases and the person will then have to restrict intake to 500 ml each day plus the previous day's output.

When the person can no longer be kept alive using conservative measures, dialysis will need to be considered. There are two main types of dialysis—peritoneal dialysis and haemodialysis.

Haemodialysis is the transfer of solutes across a semi-permeable membrane from a solution of high concentration, the blood, to one of low concentration, the dialysate. Water and small molecules, such as urea and potassium, are able to pass through the membrane.

Peritoneal dialysis

In peritoneal dialysis the peritoneum is used as a semi-permeable membrane. The peritoneum is a large area which is richly supplied with blood.

Continuous ambulatory peritoneal dialysis (CAPD), which is a practical self-dialysis method, is one of the most recent techniques for peritoneal dialysis and is the treatment of choice for many people because it permits independence from machines, a more varied diet, and a more flexible lifestyle.

A permanent indwelling catheter is inserted into the peritoneal cavity. It will become embedded by fibrous tissue which stabilizes it and minimizes leakage.

A flexible Tenckhoff catheter (Figure 12.3) is one most commonly used; it is inserted under general anaesthetic.

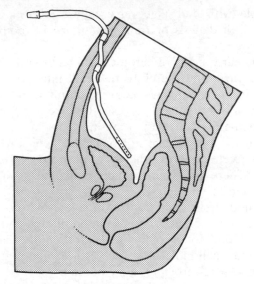

Figure 12.3 A Tenckhoff catheter in position.

Principal features of the technique

The peritoneal dialysis set, which consists of a sterile plastic bag containing the dialysate solution, is connected to the external end of the peritoneal catheter.

The dialysate bag is then raised above the person's shoulder level (Figure 12.4) and the solution is infused by gravity into the peritoneal cavity. After this, the plastic bag attached to the connecting tube is folded and placed in a pouch at the waist under the person's clothing.

At the end of the dwell/diffusion time (approximately four to five hours) the person removes the bag from the pouch unfolded and puts it near the floor (Figure 12.5) to allow the dialysis to drain by gravity.

When the dialysate is drained, a fresh bag of dialysate

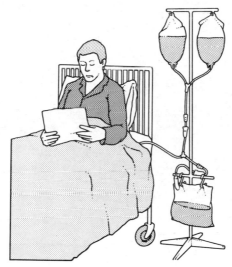

Figure 12.4 Peritoneal dialysis.

solution is attached under aseptic conditions and the procedure is repeated.

A modern technique, a 'solo disconnect CAPD system', now enables the person to disconnect the bag from connecting tubing so that only the Tenckhoff catheter is permanently attached to the body.

The most common types of peritoneal dialysis solution are 1.36% and 3.86% dextrose. The higher the concentration of dextrose, the more fluid is removed from the patient.

Most people will need to perform four to five exchanges daily and adopt their CAPD schedule to fit their daily activities, and will perform the last exchange at bedtime with a long overnight dwell period (8–10 hours). This allows the person uninterrupted sleep.

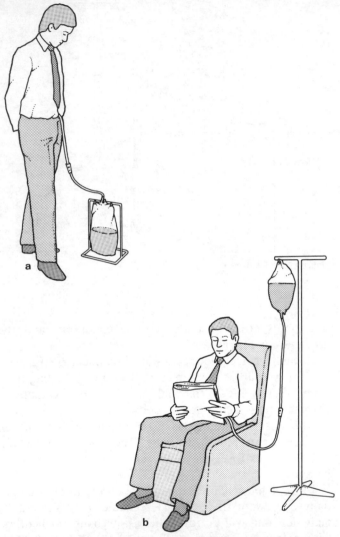

Figure 12.5 Continuous ambulatory peritoneal dialysis: (a) draining out; (b) running in.

Education/Support

The success of this method depends on the person's scrupulous attention to cleanliness.

The person must be instructed in aseptic technique when caring for the catheter. They must be able to understand and report any signs and problems which could result in peritonitis, such as:

- cloudy peritoneal fluid
- abdominal pain or tenderness
- an increase in temperature
- discharge/inflammation around the Tenckhoff catheter site

The person must keep a daily chart in which each exchange is documented, and their weight and blood pressure recorded.

Haemodialysis

In this procedure the person's blood is cleansed of waste products as it passes through an artificial kidney which is connected to a dialysis machine.

In the machine there are layers of an artificial semi-permeable membrane. The blood will pass through this artificial membrane which acts like the glomerulus in the kidney. The other side of the membrane is bathed in dialysis fluid, and the waste products from the blood diffuse into the dialysis fluid. The blood is prevented from clotting by the addition of heparin. At the end of the procedure, waste products of protein metabolism will be removed and the electrolyte and water balance will have been restored.

In order to perform regular dialysis, access to circulation must be available.

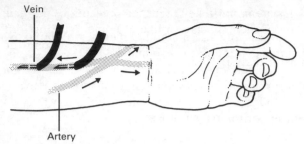

Figure 12.6   A Cimino fistula.

Methods of access

Cimino fistula

Cimino fistula (Figure 12.6) is a subcutaneous anastomosis between an artery and a vein sited usually in the arm. The vein becomes dilated, enabling needles to be introduced into an enlarged arterialized vein. These needles can then be connected to the tubing of the dialysis machine.

Grafts

Synthetic grafts are now being used in certain circumstances. The graft connects an artery to a vein, creating an arterio-venous fistula. They are usually sited in the forearm but sometimes may be used in the thigh.

Subclavian catheters

A technique has been adapted where a special subclavian catheter is inserted into a subclavian vein, enabling haemodialysis to take place. This procedure has the advantage of being fairly simple and quick to perform, which allows emergency access and person mobility.

The person will be taught the precautions that must be taken of their subclavian line at home. Nursing staff will care for the catheter site when the person comes to the unit for dialysis sessions.

Transplantation

Renal transplantation from a live or cadaver donor is an alternative to dialysis in end-stage renal failure and gives the person a chance to live a more normal life. Steroid and immunosuppressive drugs are used to combat rejection and are taken for life. Survival rates are between 70 and 80% at one year compared with 90% or more after one year on dialysis.

Each individual is assessed physically and emotionally to determine their ability to cope with living with a chronic illness.

Terminal care

If a person with end-stage renal failure is not able to have dialysis or transplantation there will come a time when conservative methods of treatment fail.

It is of utmost importance to relieve the unpleasant problems of uraemia such as vomiting and chest pain. An anti-emetic drug, e.g. prochlorperazine, can be given in conjunction with diamorphine.

Oral fluids are given as required, as the person is usually very thirsty and has an unpleasant taste in the mouth. Mouth care should be performed at least two-hourly and the person's position should be changed frequently.

The relatives should be kept completely informed and encouraged to help with the person's care.

Death often occurs suddenly as a result of the high serum potassium causing cardiac arrest.

POLYCYSTIC KIDNEYS

This is a hereditary progressive cystic condition of both kidneys causing chronic renal failure in middle age. The kidneys become very large with multiple cysts. It causes episodes of haematuria and loin pain. The person will eventually require dialysis or transplantation. Bilateral nephrectomy is sometimes indicated because of chronic infection in the cysts.

RENAL CALCULI

Stones may form in the renal tract. These stones are usually formed of calcium salts. Predisposing factors are:

Excessive loss of water by sweating
Urinary tract infection or stasis
Increased excretion of calcium, e.g. in metabolic disorders, prolonged bed-rest, excess of calcium in the diet

Renal colic occurs when the stone enters the ureter. The conservative treatment of renal colic is to give the person three litres of fluid in 24 hours. The urine is sieved and any stones found are sent for biochemical assay.

Analgesia, e.g. pethidine, is required. If the person fails to pass the stone, surgical intervention will be necessary.

HYPERNEPHROMA

Hypernephroma is the most common carcinoma affecting the kidney. The person presents with pain in the loin and haematuria. Metastatic deposits occur, especially in the lungs. Nephrectomy is necessary and this is followed by deep X-ray or cytotoxic therapy.

TUBERCULOSIS OF THE KIDNEY

Tuberculosis of the kidney is always secondary to a primary infection in the lungs. The person presents with frequency, dysuria and loin pain. Early morning urine specimens are cultured for acid-fast becilli (tubercle bacilli). Antituberculous therapy is commenced (see page 138).

FURTHER READING

CATTO, G. R. D. & POWER, D. A. (1988). *Nephrology in Clinical Practice*. Edward Arnold, London.

CAMERON, S. (1986). *Kidney Disease, the Facts*, 2nd edn. Oxford University Press, Oxford.

GABRIEL, R. (1980). *A Patient's Guide to Dialysis and Transplantation*. MTP, Lancaster.

GABRIEL, R. (1988). *Renal Medicine*, 3rd edn. Baillière Tindall, London.

GOODLINSON, S. (1984). Renal function, an overview. *Nursing*, **2**, 843, 845–846, 848, 851–852.

GOODLINSON, S. & HOLMES, S. (1985). Acute renal failure, aetiology and emergency treatment. *Nursing*, **2**, 1254–1257.

HOLMES, S. (1984). The nutritional management of renal disease. *Nursing*, **2**, 860–862.

LEIGH. J. (1985). Acute renal failure. *Nursing*, **2**, 1258–1259.

MURPHY, A. (1989). Renal dialysis—Concepts and principles. *Nursing Review*, **7**(2), 3–4.

NORRIS, M. K. G. (1989). About acute renal failure. *Nursing*, **19**(6), 21.

ULDALL, R. (1987). *Renal Nursing*, 3rd edn. Blackwell Scientific, Oxford.

13 Nursing people with problems of their nervous system

The nervous system is the control and communication system of the body. It is responsible for receiving and interpreting the messages which the body receives from its environment, for conscious sensation, and for control of motor activity. Disorders of the nervous system manifest themselves by changes in motor control, sensory perception, in consciousness or in behaviour.

NERVE TISSUE

Nerve tissue is made up of millions of nerve cells or neurones and their processes. These are the functional units of the nervous system and are supported by connective tissue cells called glial cells.

Neurones

Nerve cells vary in size and shape but each has a cell body which contains a nucleus embedded in protoplasm. Each neurone has many processes: the short ones are called dendrites and the long process is called the axon or nerve fibre (Figure 13.1).

Impulses are transmitted from one neurone to another by the passage of a small electrical current down the axon from the cell body. This is produced by the movement of sodium and potassium ions across the membrane of the axon. When the current reaches the end of the axon, a

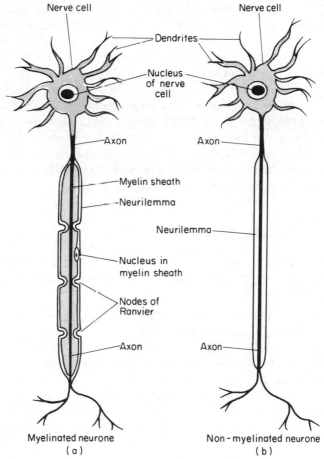

Figure 13.1 A neurone.

neurotransmitter chemical is released. These chemicals cross the synapse between the processes of the cells and either stimulate or inhibit the next cell in producing its own electrical current.

In some neurones, the axon is insulated by a myelin membrane. In order that impulses may be transmitted along myelinated nerve fibres, the myelin sheath is absent at certain points known as the nodes of Ranvier. The impulses pass from one node of Ranvier to the next.

White matter refers to aggregations of myelinated axons from many neurones, supported by neurological cells. The lipid substance myelin has a whitish colour that gives the white matter its name.

Grey matter is the part of the nervous system which contains either nerve cell bodies and dendrites or bundles of unmyelinated axons and neurological cells.

THE NERVOUS SYSTEM

The nervous system is composed of the central nervous system, the peripheral nervous system and the autonomic nervous system.

The central nervous system

The central nervous system comprises the brain and the spinal cord.

The brain can be anatomically divided into three parts: the cerebrum, the cerebellum and the brain stem (which includes the midbrain, the pons and the medulla oblongata). The brain occupies the interior of the skull and is continuous with the spinal cord at the foramen magnum (the hole in the base of the skull through which the spinal cord passes).

The spinal cord runs in the spinal canal from the foramen magnum to the level of the first lumbar vertebra. Although anatomically the spinal cord is a continuous structure, it is convenient to divide the cord into eight cervical, twelve thoracic, five lumbar, five sacral and one coccygeal segment. Each segment receives sensory (afferent) nerve roots and gives off motor (efferent) nerve roots on either side. These nerve roots join together to form peripheral nerves which pass out between the vertebrae.

The brain and spinal cord are covered by protective membranes called meninges. These are the:

Dura mater—outer layer
Periosteal layer
– Arachnoid mater—middle layer
– Pia mater—inner layers

The peripheral nervous system

The peripheral nervous system comprises the sympathetic system and the parasympathetic system. The nerve fibres of these systems are non-myelinated (see Figure 13.1b) and are concerned mainly with the control of involuntary muscle. They consist largely of efferent neurones: motor fibres supplying the involuntary muscles in the walls of organs such as the stomach, intestines, bladder, heart and blood vessels, and secretory fibres supplying organs such as the liver, pancreas and kidney.

INVESTIGATIONS

Plain X-rays

Skull, spinal and chest X-rays may be performed.

Electroencephalography (EEG)

The electrical activity of the brain can be measured and compared with a normal pattern.

Lumbar puncture

A lumbar puncture is frequently performed in neurological diseases:

- To remove a sample of cerebrospinal fluid (CSF) for diagnostic purposes.
- To estimate and perhaps reduce cerebrospinal pressure.
- To give drugs (intrathecal injections)
- To introduce radiological contrast

A needle is usually inserted between the third and fourth lumbar vertebrae so as to prevent damage to the spinal cord. Following the procedure the person is advised to lie flat to prevent headaches which may develop due to low pressure. It is also important to encourage a fluid intake of 200 ml hourly to help the formation of cerebrospinal fluid.

Cerebral angiography

The cerebral blood vessels can be shown by injecting a radio-opaque contrast medium into the carotid artery. This investigation can be performed under general anaesthesia. It is important to observe the puncture site and monitor the neurological state of the person for six to eight hours following this procedure.

Computerized axial tomography (CAT scan, CT scan)

This is an invaluable non-invasive investigation which involves a series of X-ray tomograms cutting through the brain from the occiput upwards. The contents of the skull are visualized and a computerized assessment can be made of the density of the structures X-rayed. This technique has largely superseded cerebral angiography and pneumoencephalography.

Nuclear magnetic resonance scanning (NMR)

This is a non-invasive investigation which measures the absorption and re-emission of units of energy from atoms. It gives clear pictures of tissues without the need to introduce a radioactive substance into the body. The procedure is similar to a CAT scan.

Myelography

A myelography is a radiological examination in which a contrast solution is used to outline the subarachnoid space, the spinal cord and its nerve roots. It is used to delineate tumours of the spine and prolapsed inter-vertebral discs. The patient will have to lie flat or sit upright according to which contrast medium is used.

Visual field testing

The nerve fibres from the retina of the eye pass through the optic nerves, the optic chiasma and the optic tracts to the visual cortex in the occipital lobe. Changes in the integrity of this pathway may lead to defects in the patient's field of vision.

Electromyography (EMG)

Electrical activity occurs within the muscle fibres and can be detected by needle electrodes inserted into the muscles.

Digital vascular imaging (DVI)

This is an examination of the vascular system which permits angiography, without the use of catherers, simply by the intravenous injection of contrast medium. It is combined with electronic and computer technology.

NURSING ASSESSMENT OF NEUROLOGICALLY IMPAIRED PEOPLE

Neurological assessment of the person by the nurse is of vital importance, as the interpretation of these observations will give the first indication of the improvement or deterioration of the person's condition.

This assessment will be recorded on a neurological observation chart, and the one that has come into universal use is the Glasgow Coma Scale. The advantage of this chart is that all the terms used will have the same meaning to all nursing and medical staff (see Figure 13.2). Using a neurological observation chart will indicate how the person's conscious level is functioning. Recordings are evaluated in three sections. These are:

- Eye opening
- Verbal response
- Motor response

The person is given a score for the best response that they can achieve. These observations will indicate what ability the person has to hear, appreciate and obey instructions.

Pupils

The third cranial nerve controls the pupils ability to constrict and when injury causes the brain to become oedematous the pressure will build up because the skull cannot expand. This increasing pressure pushes on the brain which also compresses the third cranial nerve. Pupils are normally round and equal and react to light. They must be checked for size, shape and reaction to light. When light is shone directly in one eye, that pupil should constrict; this is the direct light reflex. At the same time, the pupil of the other eye should also constrict; this is

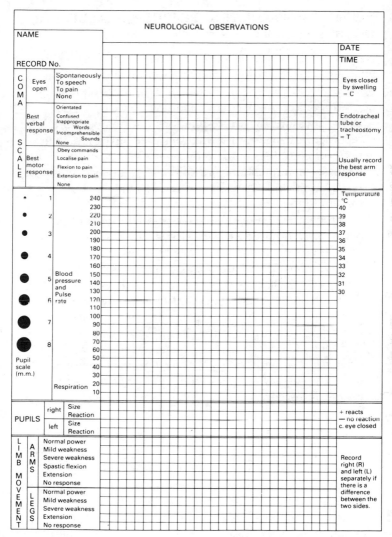

Figure 13.2 Glasgow Coma Scale

called a consensual reflex. Pupil changes are often late signs of increasing pressure within the skull.

A change in the level of consciousness is the first sign of rising intracranial pressure.

Vital signs

Blood pressure, pulse, respirations and temperature are recorded. Changes in the vital signs are also a late indication of neurological deterioration. When there is an increase in intracranial pressure the brain becomes hypoxic, so the blood pressure increases to try and get more oxygen to the brain.

If the intracranial pressure is equal to or higher than the blood pressure, death will occur. Increased pressure on the vaso-motor centre leads to slowing of the pulse (bradycardia). Respiratory impairment is not uncommon. Temperature changes may be seen if there is pressure on the temperature control mechanism in the hypothalamus.

A high temperature is damaging to a person with increased pressure because it increases the metabolic demands of the brain, thereby increasing the workload. Chemical transmitters work at an optimum temperature of 37°C; a higher temperature may disrupt pathways and lead to fits occurring.

Limb movements

Our voluntary movements are controlled by nerve tracts (cortico-spinal) and these tracts originate in the brain. Any lesion in the brain putting pressure on these tracts will cause deficits in our limb movements.

When the nurse checks for limb movements, they should look at the position of limbs, and check that they are equal.

Paresis (weakness) or plegia (paralysis) is an important

sign. Strength of the extremities should be tested. To test the limbs in the upper extremity the person may be asked to squeeze the nurse's fingers. If they squeeze each of the nurse's hands at the same time the nurse may feel some difference in strength, but this can be inaccurate as with many people their dominant hand is always stronger.

The other method to test the strength of the arms is to ask the person to hold both arms outstretched in front of their body, palms up, fingers stretched and eyes closed; after a short period the weak arm will waver and gradually fall downwards.

To test lower extremity strength the person must be asked to raise their legs up off the bed and push the sole of the foot against the nurse's hand. It is important to compare each side and to record the difference between right and left limbs and changes in the responses of an individual limb.

The key point to remember is that it is change in the recordings that are important and which must be reported.

CEREBRO-VASCULAR ACCIDENT

Oxygen and glucose are the two essential requirements for cerebral metabolism and a continual blood supply is essential. The brain receives its blood from four main arteries, the two internals and the two vertebral arteries.

The conducting arteries and the areas they supply are:

1. Internal carotid arteries—most of the cerebral hemispheres and the basal ganglia
2. Vertebral arteries—the brain stem, the cerebellum and the occipital lobe.

These two systems anastomose or meet at the circle of Willis (Figure 13.3).

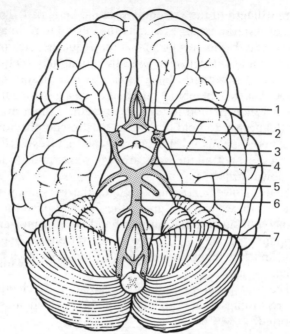

Figure 13.3   The circle of Willis. 1, anterior cerebral artery; 2, middle cerebral artery; 3, internal carotid artery; 4, posterior communicating artery; 5, posterior cerebral artery; 6, basilar artery; 7, vertebral artery.

There is a group of disorders, and the problems are due to the insufficiency of the blood supply to the brain. The three main causes of reduced blood supply to the brain are vascular:

Cerebral haemorrhage
Cerebral thrombosis
Cerebral embolism

Following a CVA an area of the brain will be deprived of its blood supply, resulting in necrosis. When this happens there will be a loss of voluntary movement on the opposite side of the body.

CVA is the most frequent neurological disorder of adults. Only a third of those who suffer this are able to return to a fully functioning life.

A CVA is commonly known as a stroke. Conditions which may predispose a patient developing a CVA are:

– Cardiac diseases
– Diabetes
– Hypertension
– Cigarette smoking

Cerebral haemorrhage

This is associated with atherosclerosis which causes degeneration of the arterial walls, and commonly follows a long history of hypertension.

Most people experience a very severe headache with or without vomiting which may be followed by loss of consciousness.

A large haemorrhage coupled with a loss of consciousness has a poor prognosis; approximately half of those affected die within a few days.

Cerebral thrombosis

Cerebral thrombosis is associated with atherosclerosis in which the lumen of the artery is narrowed, slowing down the blood flow and leading to the formation of thrombi. Once the vessel becomes occluded, the area of cerebral tissue it supplied becomes necrotic.

A CVA which has been caused by thrombosis is seen most often in the elderly. Many of the elderly tend to have a history of diabetes or hypertension.

The onset of a thrombosis tends to occur during sleep

or soon after rising. This is thought to be related to the fact that elderly people have decreased sympathetic activity, and recumbancy causes a lowering of blood pressure which can lead to brain ischaemia.

Cerebral embolism

This is often a piece of thrombus which has broken free and is circulating on its own. A cerebral embolism is frequently the result of heart disease.

A thrombus within the heart may break up and fragments enter the circulation. A cerebral embolism may also occur as a result of a fat embolism following a fracture of a femur or pelvis. This is frequently of sudden onset.

Problems resulting from a cerebrovascular accident

The problems of a CVA are varied. They depend on the condition causing the stroke and the size and location of the area of the brain tissue affected by the vascular accident. Onset may vary from gradual to sudden.

1. Level of consciousness may range from an unconscious to a conscious state.
2. Those in a conscious state complain of severe headache and vomiting.
3. Hemiplegia (paralysis one side of the body) is common with decreased muscle tone and loss of relexes on the affected side.
4. Asphasia (loss of speech) or dysphasia (difficulty with speaking) may occur.
5. There may be some memory impairment and the person is unaware of their condition, but in many instances they will be shocked and frightened to find themselves paralysed and unable to express themself.

The aim of care in the acute phase is to prevent complications from the original CVA from the immobility it causes and the loss of function caused by focal defects.

Problem

Alteration in level of consciousness.

Actions

A change in the level of consciousness is the most sensitive indicator of improvement or deterioration.

- The level of consciousness can change from minute to minute.
- Assess the person's ability to maintain airway, swallow, cough.

Problem

Impairment of physical immobility.

Actions

- The limbs of a person with acute hemiplegia are often flaccid at first but may become spastic as muscle tone returns.
- The joints can become flexed and fixed in useless positions, with deformities like foot drop, wrist drop and contractures, unless preventative measures are taken.
- The person's limbs should be carefully placed in the normal anatomical positions to maintain good body alignment (see Figure 13.4).
- All the person's joints must be put through a range of passive movements. When the person is dependent and

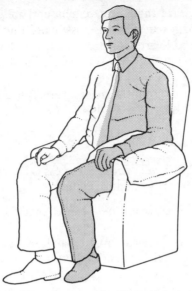

Figure 13.4 Supporting a person with a left hemiplegia in a chair.

confined to bed, their position is changed and passive movements are carried out two-hourly.
• Early mobilization, e.g. walking, is discouraged.

Problem

Impairment of communication.

Dysphasia can cause immense feelings of anger and impotence because of the difficulties in communication. The resultant loss of self-esteem, depression and frustration can cause serious problems.

Actions

• Treat the person as an intelligent adult. Talk directly to the person with sufficient light on you to enable the person to see your facial movement and body language. Phrase as many questions as possible so that the person can answer 'yes' or 'no'.

- Use gestures and other visual cues to add meaning to your words.
- Elicit responses from the person, e.g. 'please nod your head if you understand'.
- Reinforce every correct response. Keep the person's environment relaxed as far as possible.
- Keep in the social world—have family and grand-children to visit.
- Communicate empathy for the person's problem and show genuine interest.

Problem

Alteration in normal elimination patterns. Control of the bladder and bowels is behaviour that we all learn in childhood and is associated with cleanliness and growing up. One can realize how loss of this function is not only a cause of great physical distress but also of much psychological suffering.

Actions

- Assess the person's awareness of the need to micturate. Record fluid balance. Observe for signs of urinary retention.
- Assess the person's previous history of diet or constipation.

Problem

Alteration in food and fluid intake.

Actions

- With people who may be semi-comatose or who have

swallowing difficulties it may be necessary to use intravenous fluids or have a nasogastric tube passed and tube feedings commenced.

- When consciousness is regained and the person can swallow, oral feeding can be commenced with semi-solids such as ice cream (liquids are difficult to swallow initially).
- Small frequent feedings may be better tolerated than large meals; cut the person's food into bite-size pieces, and give food from the unaffected side.
- Encourage the person to feel that the problem is not overwhelming.
- Many self-help devices to help the person feed themself are available.

Problem

Susceptibility to pressure sores.

Actions

See page 39.

Problem

Unable to maintain own hygiene due to restricted body movement.

Action

Provide facilities for the person to wash themself as much as possible and only give help where needed.

Problem

Impaired social interaction.

Actions

- Try to anticipate the needs of the person and provide a safe secure environment to minimize anxiety and for the person to develop trust in the nurses.
- Rehabilitation starts as soon as the person is conscious, to ensure the maximum degree of recovery.
- The person is evaluated on the ability to carry out the activities of daily living and is assisted by the occupational therapist and physiotherapist, together with the nurse, in becoming independent in each activity as far as possible.
- As the person's independence returns, the occupational therapist will help to supervise activities such as getting in and out of the bath, dressing, feeding, and cooking. They may provide aids such as adapted cutlery, non-stick mats and aids for bathing and going to the toilet.

The social worker and occupational therapist in conjunction with the family will be involved in assessing the home situation to ensure that any problems that the person has at home could be overcome.

MULTIPLE SCLEROSIS

To link the brain with the muscles, the body employs a relay system composed of neurones. In the motor system most of these neurones are insulated with a myelin sheath. This enables nerve impulses to travel much faster along the fibre. (See Figure 13.1a.)

In myelinated fibres there are gaps in the sheath called the nodes of Ranvier, and the impulse is able to leap along the nerve fibre from node to node.

When voluntary movement occurs, two neurones, the upper motor neurone and lower motor neurone, are involved with the connection (synapse) in the spinal cord

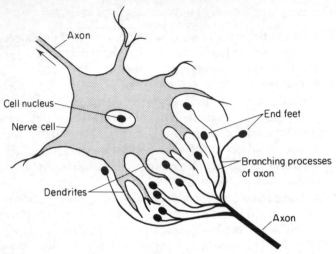

Figure 13.5   Diagram of a synapse.

(Figure 13.5). Multiple sclerosis interrupts this pathway. The cause is unknown. There are areas of sclerosis (scarring) along the myelin sheath which covers the nerve fibres, causing death of the myelin; the nerve is therefore no longer able to conduct impulses correctly. This leads to impairment of the function of the area supplied by the nerve.

The degeneration of myelin occurs only in central nerves and not in the peripheral nerves.

Invariably, disorders of movement occur, and depending on the site of the neurone, once it dies the person will be left with a paralysis of the limbs, or loss of sphincter control, or both.

As multiple sclerosis can affect any part of the central nervous system, there is a wide range of problems. A feature of this condition is its tendency to undergo remissions and relapses, and many people have little or no disability for many years after the initial diagnosis.

Early signs:
1. Weakness and sensory disturbances.
2. Visual disturbances.
   Blurring of vision diplopia.
   Double vision.
   Pain on movement of eyes.
3. Abnormal reflexes.
4. Sensation of numbness or tingling (paraesthesia) in a limb.
   Weakness of limbs.
   Common in lower limbs with dragging of foot.
   Can also involve arms with loss of power.
   Inability to perform fine movements with hands.
5. Sphincter impairment.
   Later signs:
   - Spastic paraplegia.
   - Walking becomes difficult as spasticity of legs increases.
   - Ataxia.
   (a) Due to cerebellar and brain stem lesions.
   (b) Co-ordination of hand movements difficult and characterized by a jerkiness (intention tremor).
   (c) Irregular and jerky movements of the lower limbs may occur.
   (d) Slurring of speech.
   (e) Emotional lability, euphoria, depression.

There is no cure for multiple sclerosis; the treatment is aimed at relieving problems and giving support. This increases in amount and complexity as the disease progresses.

People are usually only admitted to hospital when complete dependence has been reached or if there are secondary complications, e.g. bladder and chest infection, or if family circumstances necessitate it.

The aim of care is to keep the person as active and functional as possible in order to lead a purposeful life, to relieve the person's problems, and to provide continuing support as and when needed.

(This section on problems and actions will be confined to the care of the person in the later stages when paraplegia has occurred.)

Problem

Impaired mobility.

Muscle spasticity and weakness, especially in the lower limbs, is a common problem in multiple sclerosis.

Actions

Regular passive movements to preserve joint function and prevent muscle shortening. Contractures can start developing within 36 hours and will continue to develop unless the joints are put through a range of passive movements at regular intervals.

Problem

Susceptibility to pressure sores.

Motor involvement prevents the person from moving about easily and changing position; therefore, pressure sores can develop.

Actions

See page 39.

Problem

Risk of problems of elimination.

Actions

- Assess person's awareness of the need to micturate and its control.
- Ensure adequate fluid intake.
- Monitor and record intake and output daily.
- For people who have lost bladder control, external devices will have to be used to limit the effects of incontinence.
- Bowel function should be assessed together with the person's previous history of diet or constipation.
- A high-roughage diet, a good fluid intake and regular aperients may be required.
- Some people cannot evacuate faeces and may need suppositories or an enema before manual evacuation.

Problem

Impaired eyesight or unable to hold book.

Actions

- Talking books (Tape).
- Page-turning machines.
- Arrange the bed so that the person will be able to see people approaching.

Problem

Person may have difficulty in eating.

Actions

- Cranial nerves which mediate the articulation of swallowing are often affected, because of the person's immobility; weakness in mastication and swallowing and anxiety will lead to a very poor appetite. (Also, inhalation pneumonia can occur, and is often the cause of death.)

- Monitor food intake.
- Give meals that are easily digested.
- Supportive crockery and cutlery will help the person.
- High-calorie and blender foods may be necessary in order to meet the person's nutritional requirements.
- Suction apparatus must always be available.

Problem

Difficulty with speaking.

Actions

- The services of a speech therapist to strengthen the muscles and to improve dysarthria will be required.
- Take time to listen when the person tries to speak.

Problem

Unable to maintain own hygiene because of restricted body movement.

Action

Provide support and facilities for the person to wash themselves as much they can and then give help where needed.

Psychological care

The fact that this disease is progressive means that psychological support is critical. People whose condition is deteriorating and who can see their level of movement decreasing can become very depressed and may find it difficult to persevere with exercise.

The nursing care plan must include helping the person to be as active as possible. Efforts must be made to provide some sort of recreational activity that suits the patient. Research has looked at the effect of physical activity on sedentary females and found that those who had partaken in programmes to improve their activities gained in feelings of self-esteem and appearance. Self-help specialist support groups can be a great help to patients, not only with practical tips but also in providing experiences with similar problems, e.g. The Multiple Sclerosis Society.

EPILEPSY

In the normal brain, nerve cells function by discharging small electrical impulses. Epilepsy is thought to be due to an electrical disturbance in the nerve cells in one section of the brain that causes them to give off abnormal recurrent uncontrolled discharges which may remain localized or spread throughout the brain. Loss or impairment of consciousness with convulsions frequently occurs in association with an attack.

Epilepsy may be:

(a) Idiopathic—without known cause.
(b) Symptomatic—the problems of epilepsy may be caused by an intracranial pathological condition, e.g. cerebral tumours or head injury, or fits may occur due to hyperpyrexia, hypocalcaemia or hypoglycaemia.

The aim of treatment is to determine the underlying cause and to treat it.

Electroencephalography is the main investigation performed; it records the electrical activity of the brain and is useful in locating the site where the epileptic discharge begins. Investigative procedures such as a scan and laboratory studies are done to rule out organic lesions.

Petit mal (minor epilepsy)

Petit mal epilesy is idiopathic and usually begins in childhood. It takes the form of momentary alterations of consciousness, so that the person, for example, may pause in conversation, have a vacant expression, or suddenly stop while walking. The problem with such attacks is that they may occur in a place which may be dangerous, for example in the bath or in the middle of the road.

Temporal lobe epilepsy

In fits caused by lesions in or near the temporal lobe, the aura, which is always prominent, may be the sole feature or the attack may progress to a generalized convulsion.

A wide variety of sensory and motor disturbances may occur. Sensory disturbances take the form of hallucinations of smell, taste and perception. The latter is known as the 'deja vu' phenomenon—a feeling that what is happening has happened before. Motor disturbances are equally varied. The person looks dazed and does not respond normally when questioned. Aggressive behaviour occasionally occurs.

Jacksonian or focal epilepsy

Jacksonian epilepsy is a convulsion originating in the precentral motor cortex and is responsible for some gross postural movements. The attack starts in one part of the body and is either limited to this area or spreads, when it may progress to a major convulsion. One common pattern is for a convulsion to begin with a thumb or finger and the corner of the mouth. It progresses down that side of the body and may then involve the opposite limbs in a generalized fit with loss of consciousness.

Grand mal (major epilepsy)

It is important that the nurse should understand that when the person has an epileptic attack (grand mal fit) it may go through four stages.

The aura

This is a warning; the person will complain of a variety of sensations, e.g.

Epigastric discomfort
Vertigo
Feelings of fear

It lasts a very short time, and may give the person time to anticipate the fit and move away from obvious danger. Not all people have an aura.

Tonic phase

The person often cries out as they lose consciousness. All the muscles contract, arms flex, legs extend, as the muscles involved in respiration are affected. The person can become cyanosed. This phase may last about 5 to 30 seconds.

Clonic phase

This is the convulsing stage when the muscles repeatedly relax and contract, sometimes violently, and there may be incontinence. After about two minutes the convulsing gradually ceases and the person lapses into a flaccid coma.

Coma phase

The muscles relax, and the person's level of consciousness improves. The person may be confused and dazed, or

respond normally and then fall into a deep sleep for
several hours, waking with no memory of the seizure and
the brief conscious interlude.

The nurse must remember that people suffering a grand
mal seizure do not necessarily pass through all the stages
just described.

There is considerable individual variation in the way a
grand mal seizure manifests itself.

Nursing care will be different during a fit than when the
person is over the acute phase and ready for education
about the disorder.

During the fit the nurse stays with the person until
they are fully conscious. The observations and recording
of events are crucial for their safety, and can be a valuable
help in diagnosis and monitoring the effectiveness of
treatment.

The following observations must be made when
observing the person having an attack:

- *Onset*. Note time of onset; was it sudden or was it
  preceded by an aura? Did the person let out a cry?
- *Duration*. How long did the fit last?
- *Motor activity*. If convulsions occurred, where did they
  start, and did they spread to any other part of the body?
- *Eyes, tongue, teeth*. Were the teeth clenched or open?
  Was there any eye or tongue deviation to one side or
  turning of the head?
- Note the size and reaction of pupils.

Nursing during an attack

Problem

Has the potential for injury due to loss of consciousness
and the uncontrolled muscle contractions.

Actions

During the attack:

- Maintenance of a clear airway is crucial. If the person has their teeth clenched in spasm, do not attempt to insert the mouth gag. This can cause teeth to be broken and perhaps aspirated. Mouth gags and airways are only helpful if introduced before the teeth become clenched.
- If on the floor, place pillows, etc. under the head to reduce injury.
- Roll the person on side to aspirate if vomiting occurs.
- Loosen constrictive clothing.
- Restraining the person should not be attempted.
- If possible, provide privacy for the person and protect them from curious onlookers.

If the person is already in hospital, precautions can be taken by:

- Having the person's bed where it can easily be observed.
- Keeping the bed low.
- Suction equipment readily available.
- Always taking the person's temperature under their axilla.
- Supervising the person if they smoke.

Level of consciousness:

- Was the person unconscious, and if so how long for? On regaining consciousness was the person confused or fully aware?
- Was there any memory of the event?

Respirations:

- Observe rate, quality or absence of respirations; was the person cyanosed?

Body activity:

- Was there any incontinence (urine or faeces), vomiting, foaming at the mouth, bleeding from mouth or tongue?
- Was there any obvious paralysis or weakness of arms or legs after the attack. This is called Todd's paralysis.
- Was the person suffering from amnesia?
- Were there any other bodily injuries such as hitting the head from falling?
- When questioned does the person recall any experiences such as emotional or physical stress just before the attack?

The aim of treatment is to prevent fits so that the person with epilepsy can live as normal a life as possible.

The most common therapy is the use of anticonvulsant drugs. Anticonvulsant drugs are thought to act by increasing the stability of the neuronal membranes by altering the electrochemical ion permeability; this prevents the spread of the abnormal brain activity. Some of the commoner drugs used are:

Phenobarbitone (60–300 mg/day)
Phenytoin (150–600 mg/day)
Primidone (125–1500 mg/day)
Sodium valproate (600–2600 mg/day)
Clonazepam (1–8 mg/day)
Carbamazepine (800–1600 mg/day)

Some people may require a combination of two or more anticonvulsant drugs.

Clinical trials into a new drug Vigabatrin have shown

that treatment can cut fit frequency significantly, with half the people treated having a 50% greater reduction.

Long-term management

Aims

- To prevent the recurrence of seizures and therefore allow the person to lead a normal life.
- For the person to accept that they have epilepsy and comply with the drug therapy and the necessary modifications in their lifestyle which may be necessary.

Education of person and family

- Help the person to understand and be aware of the possible side-effects of the drugs, e.g. drowsiness, ataxia, diplopia and rashes, and to report them to the doctor or nurse for the dosage to be adjusted.
- The person must be warned about the dangers of running out of medication and of sudden cessation of the therapy.
- The person may sometimes forget to take a dose of medication; it is then best for the person to make up for this by taking an extra tablet within the same 24 hours.
- To avoid alcohol when seizures are known to follow alcoholic intake.
- Alcohol is an enzyme inducer and can increase the metabolism of anticonvulsants. Stabilized epileptics who may start to drink or stop drinking alcohol may require dosage adjustment.
- Help the person's family to understand about the seizures and what to do in case of a seizure. Families can be very frightened about seizures, due to them being unexpected and unpredictable. If they have the knowledge about what to do in case of a seizure some of the fear is removed.

- Encourage the person to study themself and their environment to determine what specific factors precipitate their seizures and therefore help to prevent them.
- The person must be informed about the help and support that can be given by the British Epilepsy Association, and must be encouraged to wear a bracelet that indicates the problem and carry a card with their doctor's name and phone number, and the medication that they are taking. The point of this is that, should a seizure occur outside the home, people will understand what is happening and the appropriate care can be given.
- Advice should be given concerning activities during which a fit would be dangerous, e.g. swimming, smoking, certain games, but many of these activities are safe as long as the person is accompanied. Showers are considered safer than baths.
- There are legal restrictions regarding driving; the person must have been free from attacks for three years before he can apply for a licence. This only applies to private cars and not to heavy goods or public service vehicles. The person is then encouraged to live as normal a life as possible despite the invisible disability.

Status epilepticus

In status epilepticus, attacks follow each other without the person regaining consciousness. It is a grave emergency and admission to the hospital is necessary. Management involves stopping the cycle of the fits by use of intravenous drugs such as diazepam, maintaining a clear airway and preventing injury. Full care of the unconscious person is necessary. Padded cot sides will be required. A common precipitating factor in status epilepticus is when a person suddenly stops taking their anticonvulsant drugs.

PARKINSON'S DISEASE

Parkinson's disease is a progressive neurological disorder affecting the brain centres responsible for the control of movement. It is associated with a decreased concentration of dopamine. Dopamine is produced by the substantia nigra (a nucleus of pigmented cells in the midbrain which functions as part of the extrapyramidal system). Dopamine is delivered to the basal ganglia via the nerve axons where it appears to be essential for the normal functioning of the basal ganglia.

Research has also shown that the level of the chemical transmitter acetylcholine within the nervous system is increased. The signs and symptoms of this disease are due to this imbalance of chemical transmitters. The cause of the disease is unknown. It affects one person out of every 1000 in the UK, with one person in every 100 in the 60–70 year age group. Men and women are affected equally.

Assessment

Tremor:

- Onset is insidious; the person hardly notices the initial shaking of the hand or foot, expecting it to pass, but is gradually distressed to realize that this tremor is most marked when resting.
- The tremor develops initially in the distal portion of the limbs and eventually involves the head, lips and tongue.
- In the upper limbs the involuntary movements are confined mainly to the wrist, fingers and tongue.
- The tremor of the fingers and thumb produce the characteristic 'pill-rolling' movement.
- A person is often embarrassed by the tremor; for example, a person may be sitting at home quietly

reading the paper and having no tremor until a visitor arrives, when a tremor may occur which the person finds socially embarrassing. They may be able to stop it by an effort of will, and will learn various tricks to stop it, e.g. holding something, sitting on the hand or stuffing their hand into a pocket.

Muscular rigidity:

- Movement of the limbs becomes jerky (cog-wheel) because of the increased muscle tone. Voluntary movements become difficult and there is a marked resistance of the limbs to passive movement.
- Even mild rigidity interferes with finely co-ordinated movements (doing up buttons, writing, etc.); generally, the person finds the rigidity more disabling than the tremor.
- The person becomes aware of muscle rigidity, not only as stiffness but as a tired aching feeling, persistent soreness or cramp. Rigidity of the head and neck is experienced as a headache, and rigidity of spinal muscles causes low back pain. Rigidity of chest muscles will cause chest pain.
- Akinesia is the inability to initiate a movement at will and impedes voluntary movement in many ways. Dressing and eating takes much longer. The person is slow to initiate walking and may take short shuffling steps, the body leans forward and the arms are held stiffly by the sides instead ot swinging normally. Once a person's pace increases they have difficulty in stopping. Once posture is achieved it is held for an abnormal length of time. The showness in initiating movement is most noticeable in the lack of gestures and facial expression (Cheshire cat smile).
- Rigidity of the facial muscles produces a mask-like appearance and eyes have a staring appearance. Speech

becomes slurred, weak and monotonous. Later on in the disease, the person may experience difficulty in the following ways:

- Chewing and swallowing.
- Respiratory muscles become weakened and the ability to cough is diminished, so predisposing the person to chest complications.
- The person will complain of dryness of the mouth, coldness of extremities and excessive secretion of saliva which may occur due to distrubance of the autonomic nervous system.

Treatment

Treatment is based on a combination of drug therapy, physical therapy, rehabilitation techniques for the person and education of the person and their family.

The aim of care is to have the person maintain independence in their accustomed role, and a relatively normal lifestyle for as long as the condition permits.

Principles behind the use of drug therapy

Drugs decrease problems but do not halt the progress of the disease. The drug regime will change as the disease progresses. The drugs are always given after food.

Drug therapy is aimed at redressing the balance in the brain between the neurotransmitters dopamine and acetylcholine.

The main drug used is levodopa (L-dopa) which is converted to dopamine in the basal ganglia; this reduces the person's tremor, muscular rigidity and bradykinesia. The side-effects of the drug must be monitored. L-dopa causes nausea and vomiting, postural hypotension, confusion and involuntary (choreo-athetoid) movements.

These side-effects may be reduced by the use of Sinemet which is a combination of levodopa and cardidopa.

Anticholinergics may be given to people with mild disability, who have a poor response or sensitivity to L-dopa, or they may be used in combination with L-dopa. They include Artane and Disipal.

Side-effects of the anticholinergic drugs are:

- Dryness of mouth.
- Blurred vision.
- Urinary retention.
- Constipation.

Antidepressants may be given to reduce the depression which frequently accompanies Parkinson's disease and the drug therapy. People may be managed at home on a drug programme until the advanced stage of the disorder causes marked disability and dependency.

In addition, there is considerable change and development of drugs for people with Parkinson's disease.

Selegiline (Eldepryl) is now licensed for use alone in early Parkinson's disease. The hope, as yet not realized, is that giving the drug as soon as the first problems appear could slow down the disease progression. Daily dosage is 10 mg, used alone or with levodopa.

Amantadine, less potent than levodopa, improves the clinical features of Parkinson's disease; it has the advantage of being relatively free of side-effects with the doses normally employed. Usual dose is 10 mg two times daily.

Trials with apomorphine have shown that people with prolonged severe problems of Parkinson's disease are able to increase their periods of mobility by up to four hours with subcutaneous apomorphine.

Research going on in America and Canada has shown that vitamin E may slow down the progression of symptoms. Epidemiological studies have suggested that people who, from early life, have eaten food containing high levels of the vitamin were less likely to develop Parkinson's disease in later life.

Also, stereotaxic surgery has recently been used to implant foetal brain cells into the basal ganglia. This treatment is essentially at an experimental stage and raises many ethical issues yet to be clarified.

Problems

Impairment of physical mobility.
Rigidity leading to difficulty in walking (shuffling gait).
Tremor.
Akinesia—difficulty in initiating movement (e.g. getting out of a chair).

Actions

- Initiate passive/active exercises to all extremities.
- Consult with the physiotherapist.
- Teach tricks to assist with mobility (e.g. rocking backwards and forwards to start walking).
- Encourage the person to have adequate rest periods to avoid fatigue and frustration.

Problem

Difficulties in activities of daily living—bathing, cleaning teeth, dressing.

Actions

- Assess the person and encourage independence as much as the person can manage.
- Only provide assistance when needed.
- Consult with the occupational therapist.

Problem

Altered body image—loss of self-esteem due to range of disabilities.

Action

- Try to dispel anxiety and explain to the person and family the expected outcomes of medication that will lead to reduction in rigidity and tremor.
- Evaluate the person's strengths and give as much responsibility as can be handled.

Problem

Impaired nutrition, Due to:

- difficulty in chewing/swallowing
- inadequate secretion clearance
- drooling
- decreased gag reflex.

Actions

- Assess swallowing.
- Determine the person's food likes and dislikes. Give semi-solid foods; avoid thin liquids. Small, frequent meals are better.
- Suction must be always available. If required, see that the person has glasses on and that dentures are always in place when eating a meal.
- Maintain the person in an upright position for all meals.
- Monitor fluid intake and output and weekly weighing to ensure adequate renal function and nutrition.

Problem

Alteration in bowel elimination. Constipation because of:

– Nausea.
– Decreased appetite.

Actions

- Increase fluid intake.
- Give food high in roughage.
- Increase mobility if possible.
- Give stool softeners, laxatives or suppositories as required.
- Assist with regular toileting.

Problem

Risk of urinary incontinence due to reduced mobility.

Action

Ensure that toilet/commode is easily available: men may have difficulty in using a urinal if they have a bad tremor.

Problem

Alteration in comfort, caused by difficulty in changing positions because of contracted muscles.
Unaccountable pain as a result of disturbed autonomic nervous system.
Excessive sweating.

Actions

- Turn frequently
- Warm baths.
- Massages.
- Frequent washes and changes of clothing.

Problem

Impairment of communication due to slowness of speech,

slurred speech, inability to move facial muscles, and difficulty in writing.

Actions

- Consult speech therapist. Give the person time when they are trying to speak. Encourage deep breaths before speaking.
- Suggest gestures and frame questions so that the person can answer yes or no. If there is difficulty with writing, suggest an electronic typewriter or word processor.

Problem

Difficulty in sleeping due to anxiety and discomfort.

Actions

See page 47.

The fact that the person's intellect has not been affected by the disorder must be kept in mind, as well as the tendency to become very self-conscious, depressed and withdrawn because of the person's appearance and limitations. The person and their family are advised to contact the national Parkinson's Disease Society to avail themselves of the services and group activities that they provide.

INFECTIONS

Infections may involve the membranes of the brain (meningitis), the substance of the brain (encephalitis) or the spinal cord (myelitis). Meningoencephalitis or meningoencephalomyelitis may occur, particularly in viral infections.

Meningitis

Acute meningitis, or more accurately acute leptomen-
ingitis, is inflammation of the pia mater and arachnoid
which inevitably involves the subarachnoid space and
cerebrospinal fluid. The infection reaches the meninges in
three main ways:

- Through a fracture in the skull.
- Extension to the meninges of a pre-existing pyogenic
  infection of one of the nasal sinuses, the middle ear or
  mastoid.
- Via the bloodstream.

Any pathogenic organism can cause this disease once the
subarachnoid space has been penetrated, but the commonest are meningococci, the pneumococci, streptococci
and staphylocci. Many viral infections such as measles and
glandular fever are associated with a mild meningitis.

Viral infections that mainly affect the meninges belong
to the enterovirus group. In meningococcal meningitis
death may occur rapidly.

Medical treatment and drug therapy

- A lumbar puncture and examination of the cerebrospinal fluid will be performed to aid in the diagnosis.
- Antibiotics are given. Penicillin in high doses is the
  antibiotic most commonly used in meningococcal and
  pneumococcal meningitis. It is given intramuscularly,
  intravenously, or occasionally intrathecally. Different
  antibiotics may be given according to which organism is
  isolated from the cerebrospinal fluid.
- Rehydration is necessary; intravenous fluid or fluid via
  a nasogastric tube may be given. (Nasogastric feeding is
  not done if the person has a fractured skull.)

- Lumbar punctures may be performed daily until the cerebrospinal fluid is sterile and the cell count normal.
- Analgesia is prescribed for headaches and may be given intramuscularly. The headaches can be severe.
- Sedation may be prescribed if the person is restless.

Problems

- Headache
  - usually the first sign.
  - increasing in severity.
  - may be diffuse or frontal.
  - often radiates down the neck into the back.
- Fever
  - normally 18–40°C.
- Photophobia (intolerance to light)
- Neck stiffness
  - neck cannot be flexed so as to bring the chin down on to the neck due to spasm of the extensor muscles of the neck.
- Kernig's sign may be present
  - an attempt to passively extend the knee with the hip fully flexed causes spasm of the hamstring muscles and pain.
- Vomiting
  - especially in the early stages.
- Convulsions
  - common in children.
  - rare in adults.
- Changes in level of consciousness
  - if the infection is severe.
  - drowsy.
  - irritable.
  - delerious.
  - may lapse into coma if untreated.

Actions

- Person is nursed in a darkened room due to the photophobia.
- Neurological observations are performed to assess the person's level of consciousness. (But not pupil reactions.)
- Temperature recordings are performed hourly to monitor the pyrexia and the effectiveness of antibiotics.
- Analgesia is given as required.
- Fluid intake and output are monitored to ensure that rehydration is adequate.
- If bacterial meningitis is present the person is barrier nursed to prevent cross-infection. (For care of the person on isolation nursing see Chapter 4.) This will be based on the health authority's infection control policy.
- Give assurance and support to reduce the fear, anxiety and loneliness which can be caused by this disease, particularly if the person needs to be isolated.
- Try to give all physical care together so as to give the person as much rest as possible.

Conclusions

Most people with meningitis recover, although some can be left with permanent deafness and blindness.

Encephalitis

Encephalitis (inflammation of the brain) is usually caused by a virus. Virus particles can reach the brain via the bloodstream or along the nerves, having first caused varying degrees of systemic disturbances. The severity of the disease varies according to the type of virus involved.

Acute infections are usually caused by viruses that primarily invade the brain, such as poliomyelitis or rabies.

The herpes simplex virus is responsible for many of the severe forms of encephalitis occurring in Britain. Less serious forms of encephalitis occur in diseases such as measles or mumps or occasionally as a result of vaccination, e.g. rubella vaccination.

Assessment

Headache
Mild fever
Confusion
Drowsiness
Convulsions, particularly in young children
Neck stiffness may or may not be present
Kernig's sign

Medical investigations and treatment

- There is, as yet, no specific treatment for most types of encephalitis.
- Analgesia is given for headaches.
- Lumbar punctures are performed.
- Antiviral drugs such as cytosine arabinoside may be given.
- Anticonvulsants may be required.

Actions

- Observations for convulsions is important.
- Isolation nursing may be required. (See Chapter 4).

Myelitis

Myelitis is inflammation of the spinal cord, normally involving both the grey and white matter. It may be due to a variety of causes, including bacterial infection (pyogenic or tuberculous), viral infection, and some forms of demyelinating disease.

The poliovirus is an enterovirus which affects the cells of the somatic efferent columns. It is spread by the faecal–oral route, and although rare in Britain, is still present world-wide. Immunization with live, attenuated virus taken orally on a sugar lump is greatly reducing the world incidence of the disease.

Assessment

Fever
Pain in back
– often a marked feature.
Paralysis of the trunk and lower limbs
Sensory loss
– may not be complete.
Poor control of function of the bladder and bowel

Intervention

- If a specific cause can be determined, appropriate action can be taken. This often involves a course of antibiotic therapy. If an organism cannot be isolated, a course of broad-spectrum antibiotics is prescribed.
- Nursing care is based on the degree of paralysis; the full range of nursing care with someone with paraplegia may be necessary.
- The prognosis is dependent on the nature and severity of the infection. There may be a full recovery, but permanent paralysis may occur. Even if the disease remits, concern is still present as it may have been the first sign of multiple sclerosis.

DISEASES OF THE PERIPHERAL NERVES

Peripheral neuritis means inflammation of a nerve, but the term is used generally to describe pain and impairment of the functions of a peripheral nerve. The peripheral neuropathies are a large group of diseases which can be classified into two groups—acute and chronic.

Acute neuropathy

Acute neuropathies can be classified according to the cause into acute toxic polyneuritis, acute infections, polyneuritis or acute postinfective polyneuritis (Guillain-Barré syndrome). They may:

- follow infections with known viruses, such as mumps and herpes zoster.
- result from glandular fever.
- be caused by porphyria, a disorder of haemoglobin metabolism in which episodes of haemoglobin breakdown occur.

Assessment

Prior to developing weakness, the person may have been in good health, although they may recall having had a cold or bout of 'flu'.

Numbness and weakness of all limbs
- develops rapidly over 24–48 hours.
- legs usually affected first.
- weakness spreads up the body (ascending paralysis).
Weakness of muscles of swallowing and respiration
- in severe cases.
Sensory loss
- in area of motor weakness.
Disturbed bowel and bladder function

Problem

Respiratory function must be maintained. In severe cases artificial ventilation may be required.

Action

Respiratory rate and depth are monitored. Restlessness must be noted as it may mean that cerebral hypoxia is occurring.

Problem

Risk of dehydration.

Action

Record intake and output to monitor hydration. Intravenous fluid may be required to maintain an adequate fluid intake.

Problem

Risk of joint stiffness and contractures developing.

Action

Person to have passive limb movements at least four times daily, to prevent joint stiffness and contractures. Night splints may be required. Hydrotherapy may also be used, and a bed cradle is advisable.

Problem

Person anxious and fearful because of the loss of movement and the suddenness with which it has developed.

Action

Give assurance and support as much as possible.

Other problems may include:

Risk of developing constipation.

Retention of urine is common.
Risk of developing problems of bed-rest.

Actions

See Chapter 3.

Conclusion

Acute peripheral neuropathy varies in severity and course. In most people the weakness increases for one to two weeks, then remains stationary for two to four weeks before a gradual recovery takes place. It is common for people to be in hospital for approximately two or three months. Steroids may be prescribed although their benefit is not proven.

Chronic neuropathies

There are a variety of chronic diseases which can cause peripheral neuropathy. These include carcinoma of most organs, diabetes mellitus, hypothyroidism, acromegaly, liver failure, leprosy and some hereditary diseases such as Charcot–Marie–Tooth disease.

Factors other than disease can also cause peripheral neuropathy, including industrial substances (e.g. lead, organic solvents and organic phosphates) and certain drugs (e.g. phenytoin, isoniazid and vincristine), and alcohol B_6 deficiency may occur with people who have a vegan diet.

FURTHER READING

BANKS, S. A. (1990). Consider the mind as well as the body. Nursing care and support in multiple sclerosis. *Professional Nurse*, **6**, Issue 1, 9–14.

BANKS, S. A. (1990). Multiple Sclerosis—The unpredictable enemy. *Professional Nurse*, **5**, Issue 2, 578–580.

BICKERSTAFF, E. R. (1978). *Neurology*, 3rd edn. Hodder and Stoughton, London.

DUVOISIN, R. C. (1990). *Parkinson's Disease, a Guide for the Patient and Family*, 3rd edn. Raven Press, New York.

JOHNSTONE, M. (1987). *The Stroke Patient, a Team Approach*, 3rd edn. Churchill Livingstone, Edinburgh.

LAIDLAW, W. V. & LAIDLOW T. (1984). *People with Epilepsy, How They Can be Helped*. Churchill Livingstone, Edinburgh.

LANNON, M. C. (1986). Comprehensive care of the patient with Parkinson's Disease. *Journal of Neuroscience Nursing*, **18**, No. 3, 121–131.

MYCO, F. (1983). *Nursing Care of the Hemiplegic Stroke Patient*. Harper and Row, London.

PODURGIEL, M (1990). The unconscious experience. A pilot study. Experiences of being unconscious and communicating with the unconscious patient. *Journal of Neuroscience Nursing*, **22**(1), 7–11.

PURCHESE, G. & ALLEN, D. (1984). *Neuro-medical and Neuro-surgical Nursing*, 2nd edn. Baillière Tindall, London.

REDFERN S. (1990). Care after a stroke—using Orems model. *Nursing: The journal of clinical practice, education and management*, **4**(4), 711.

RHODES, K. (1990). Parkinson's disease using the Roper model. *Nursing Times*, **86**, No. 21.

WAIN, M. E. (1986). Cerebral thrombosis. Assessment and nursing management of the acute phase. *Journal of Neuroscience Nursing*, **18**, No. 1, 31–38.

14   Nursing people with problems of their endocrine system

The endocrine glands secrete chemical substances called hormones directly into the bloodstream. These hormones are then carried to other tissues of the body where they stimulate or depress metabolic processes. In this chapter the following endocrine glands will be considered:

pituitary
thyroid
parathyroids
pancreas
adrenals

Their positions in the body are shown in Figure 14.1.

THE PITUITARY GLAND

The pituitary gland lies in a hollow in the sphenoid bone at the base of the skull. It is stimulated by the hypothalamus of the brain. The hypothalamus regulates the amount of hormones secreted by the pituitary into the blood.

The pituitary gland consists of an anterior and a posterior lobe. The *anterior lobe* produces growth hormone (GH), thyroid stimulating hormone (TSH), adrenocorticotrophic hormone (ACTH), prolactin and the gonadotrophic hormones. The *posterior lobe* produces oxytocin and antidiuretic hormone (ADH, vasopressin).

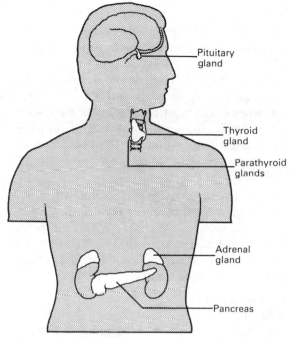

Figure 14.1 Position of the endocrine glands.

Dwarfism

Dwarfism is caused by a deficiency of growth hormone in early life. The person is normal in all respects except stature. Injection of human growth hormone will stimulate growth and enable the child to reach a normal height. The psychological effects of dwarfism are enormous; the child should be encouraged to participate in social activities which are in accordance with their age.

Gigantism

Gigantism is caused by hypersecretion of growth hormone in childhood. This is usually due to a tumour (adenoma) of the pituitary gland. If left untreated the individual can grow to 2–2.5 m (7–8 ft) tall. Pressure from the adenoma can cause headaches, vomiting and blindness. Treatment is the removal of the pituitary gland. Replacement of one or more of the hormones normally secreted by the gland may be necessary after surgery.

Acromegaly

Acromegaly is caused by hypersecretion of growth hormone in an adult, after fusion of the epiphyses of the long bone. Bone thickens, especially that of the hands, feet and skull. Facial disfiguration may occur and speech may be affected. Acromegaly is due to a tumour of the pituitary gland. Methods of treatment include:

Radioactive implants
Radiotherapy
Hypophysectomy (removal of the pituitary gland)
Cryosurgery (liquid nitrogen freezing)
Drugs (bromocriptine reduces the levels of growth hormone)

After treatment, replacement therapy with thyroxine, cortisone, oestrogen or testosterone may be necessary.

The person with acromegaly may have become very embarrassed about their altered appearance and will therefore need much psychological support from the nurse.

Simmond's syndrome

Simmond's syndrome is atrophy or destruction of the anterior lobe of the pituitary gland. The causes are infarction resulting from postpartum haemorrhage, tumour, trauma, infection or surgical removal. Problems include weakness, weight loss, amenorrhoea, atrophy of the genital organs and loss of axillary and pubic hair.

Fludrocortisone, thyroxine and oestrogen or testosterone are used as replacement therapy.

Diabetes insipidus

Diabetes insipidus is characterized by the persistent excretion of excessive quantities of urine of low specific gravity and by constant thirst, and is due to undersecretion of antidiuretic hormone (ADH, vasopressin). Causes include damage to the posterior pituitary from tumour, surgery, trauma (e.g. fractured base of skull) or idiopathic malfunction.

Assessment

Polyuria   excessive quantities of urine (5–20 l)
             – low specific gravity (1000–1004)
Dehydration – thirst
             – dry tongue
             – inelastic skin
Electrolyte imbalance

Problems

Dehydration and polyuria due to undersecretion of antidiuretic hormone.

Actions

- Assist in maintaining fluid and electrolyte balance.
- Monitor intravenous infusion.
- Record fluid intake and output.
- Assess specific gravity of urine.

- Frequent mouthwashes to keep the mouth clean and moist.
- Assess for risk of decubitus ulcers due to inelastic skin.

Replacement therapy is started with a synthetic vasopressin derivative (Pitressin) as a nasal spray or by injection. This drug treatment must continue for life. The nurse will need to educate the person about the need to always take their medication and how to use the nasal spray.

THE THYROID GLAND

The thyroid gland is situated in the neck, in association with the larynx and trachea at the level of the fifth, sixth and seventh cervical and the first thoracic vertebrae. It is a highly vascular organ. It consists of two lobes which are joined by a narrow portion called the isthmus.

It manufactures thyroid hormones which are released into the bloodstream as the body requires them. These hormones—triiodothyronine (T3) and thyroxine (T4)—control the basal metabolic rate of the body and are essential for normal mental and physical development and the functioning of the nervous system. Production of thyroid hormones is controlled by a thyroid stimulating hormone released by the anterior part of the pituitary gland. The release of this hormone is controlled by the hypothalamus.

The manufacture of thyroid hormones by the follicular cells within the thyroid gland is dependent on the presence of iodine in the body. Iodine is obtained from a variety of foods, especially sea foods and drinking water. In all continents there are regions where the soil is deficient in iodine. This will manifest itself among the inhabitants by the enlargement of the thyroid gland to form a goitre.

People can develop problems due to an overactive thyroid gland—hyperthyroidism (thyrotoxicosis)—or an underactive thyroid gland—hypothyroidism (myxoedema).

Hyperthyroidism

The cause of hyperthyroidism is not clearly understood. It is thought to be due to the activity of autonomous nodules and the stimulation of thyroid activity by thyroid stimulating immunoglobulins.

As the thyroid hormones control the body's basal metabolic rate, a wide number of problems may be present.

Assessment

Weight loss—although the person has a good appetite.
Anxiety— irritability, restlessness and fine tremor.
Heat intolerance—warm, moist skin and increased sweating.
Weakness due to muscle wasting (thyrotoxic myopathy)
Increased heart rate—tachycardia, raised blood pressure and cardiac arrythmias may be present.
Shortness of breath
Diarrhoea
Amenorrhoea, reduced sex drive and impotence can occur

In addition the person may have developed exophthalmus. This is where the eyelids retract and so the person appears to have protruding eyeballs.

Problem

Anxiety and restlessness.

Actions

- Select a quiet, unstressful area of the ward. Establish an understanding for the nursing actions required so that the person does not become unnecessarily irritable.
- Ensure clear explanation to the person and their family of the cause of the anxiety.
- Reduce other stresses, as far as is possible, in the person's and their family's lives.
- Be aware, as a nurse, of the reason for the anxiety and irritability.

Problem

Alteration in nutrition and decreased body weight.

Actions

- High-calorie, high-protein and high-carbohydrate diet. The aim is to prevent tissue breakdown caused by the high metabolic rate and to satisfy the person's increased appetite.
- Involve the dietician so as to ensure that adequate nutrition, of food the person likes, is being provided.
- Provide food in between meals.
- Fluid intake should be three to four litres daily. Excessive sweating may have caused dehydration. Explain the importance of maintaining this fluid intake.
- Weigh the person twice a week.

Problem

Exhaustion and tiredness.

Actions

- Ensure that rest is practical. Reduce activity. The

person's nervousness makes this difficult and some form of interest or distraction can help.

- Assist with sleep at night. A quiet, undisturbed environment should be provided. Aids to sleeping should be assessed, e.g. hot drinks. Sedation can be required.
- Assist with activities of daily living that cause the person fatigue.

Problem

The person may find heat uncomfortable and/or intolerable.

Actions

- Ensure limited and light bed clothing.
- Ensure that heating is turned off by the person.
- Be aware of how the person feels in response to heat and warmth.

Problem

Potential for damage to both skin and eyes.

Actions

- Assess skin for risk of decubitus ulcers. Ensure daily washing and careful drying of skin. Provide fresh, clean bed linen. Report any signs of redness or damage to the skin.
- If the person has exophthalmus, then the eyes should be protected by sunglasses. 'Eye drops may be required.

Problem

Need for knowledge about the problems caused by an overactive thyroid gland.

Actions

Assess knowledge and plan the education required for the person and their family. Areas of knowledge will need to be considered in relation to:

– Effects of the disease.
– Importance of diet.
– Reasons for anxiety and restlessness.
– Maintenance of drug therapy.
– Alternative ways of treating the problem that may be required.

There are three main approaches to the treatment of an overactive thyroid gland. These are drug therapy, radiation therapy and surgery.

Drug therapy

The drug most commonly used to control an overactive thyroid gland is carbimazole. This works primarily by interfering with the synthesis of the thyroid hormones. If people are sensitive to this drug, then propylthiouracil may be given. In addition they may require drug therapy to control problems resulting from cardiac and blood pressure changes.

Radiation therapy

People may be treated with the administration of a radioactive iodine (iodine-131). This is given orally and the radioactive iodine is trapped in the thyroid, where its radiation destroys tissue. Improvement is usually evident within three weeks and the metabolic rate should return to normal in two to three months.

This is not normally given to people who are likely to want children and never to anyone who is pregnant. There

is a danger that the thyroid gland can be reduced too far
and so a thyroxine preparation may be required.

Surgery

If these approaches are not considered advisable then
surgery may be required. The particular problems that can
occur are due to the location of the gland in relation to the
trachea, larynx and laryngeal nerves, the vascularity of the
thyroid gland and the location of the parathyroid glands
with their role in serum calcium control.

Hypothyroidism

Hypothyroidism is due to undersecretion of thyroxine. As
a result the body has a decrease in its metabolic rate. The
causes for this occurring include: congenital failure of
thyroid development, iodine deficiency, auto-immune
problems (Hashimoto's disease), following treatment for
hyperthyroidism or as a reaction to some drugs such as
lithium.

   As with hyperthyroidism, as the basal metabolic rate of
the body is altered, a number of problems may occur.

Assessment

Increased weight—although a person has a poor appetite.
Low blood pressure and cardiac rate. Cardiac
   enlargement can occur.
Dyspnoea. Pericardial and pleural effusions may have
   developed.
Dry thickened skin.
Sensitivity to cold.
Weakness and fatigue.
Dulled mental processes, with a low mood and
   depression. This can be combined with prolonged
   periods of sleep.

Menorrhagia, amenorrhoea and a low sex drive may be present.

In children, retardation of growth will occur.

The approach to people with an underactive thyroid gland is to use drug treatment. L-Thyroxine can be given, which is long-acting, and so replaces the thyroxine that the body requires. This drug needs to be taken for life. If complications occur, such as ischaemic heart disease, then triiodothyronine (T3) may be given.

Nursing actions will need to be planned in relation to the particular problems that the person is suffering from. However, the problems should resolve as the drug treatment becomes effective.

Lack of knowledge and the need for explanation

The nurse has a particular role in providing education, about the problems resulting from the disease and the need for lifelong drug treatment.

It is important that the family understands that the person's lethargy, low mood and slowness are the result of the disease, and not related to the individual's personality. There may be a need for sensitivity and patience while the drug therapy is becoming effective. In addition, the need to continue taking the drugs prescribed must be stressed. As a person feels better, there can be a tendency for them to believe that they no longer require their drugs.

THE PARATHYROID GLANDS

There are four parathyroid glands, situated in the neck behind the thyroid gland. These glands secrete para-thyroid hormone (parathormone) which helps to regulate calcium and phosphate levels in the body.

Hyperparathyroidism

Causes of overactive parathyroid glands are referred to as primary or secondary. Primary causes are normally due to a benign tumour (an adenoma). The increase in parathormone causes calcium to be withdrawn from the bones and deposited in other parts of the body, such as the renal and gastrointestinal tracts. Surgical treatment is required.

Secondary hyperparathyroidism occurs as a compensatory mechanism of the gland as a result of a decrease in the level of calcium which occurs in some diseases. This is normally treated with oral vitamin D (dihydrotachysterol).

Assessment

Lethargy and fatigue due to muscle weakness.
Anorexia.
Polyuria.
Pain
– Abdominal pain due to calcium deposits in gut and kidneys.
– Loin pain.
– Bone pain.
Fractures can occur.

Hypoparathyroidism

An underactive parathyroid gland may result in tetany. The causes of the gland being underactive include: injury, accidental removal during surgery and disease to the gland.

Assessment

Muscle twitching.

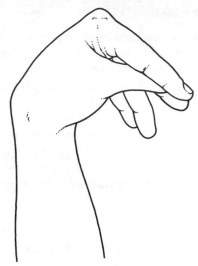

Figure 14.2   Flexion of the wrist and knuckles in hypoparathyroidism.

Tingling sensations.
Flexion of the wrist and knuckles (see Figure 14.2)
Laryngeal spasm.
Stridor.
Obstruction.
Convulsions.

Depression and psychoses can also occur.

Medical treatment

Care is aimed at relieving the tetany. This is an emergency and is done by the intravenous administration of calcium gluconate. Surgery, or maintenance doses of vitamin D (calciferol) may also be required.

THE PANCREAS

The endocrine function of the pancreas is largely concerned with the maintenance of the homeostasis of glucose within the body. Two main hormones are involved in this mechanism: glucagon, which is produced from the alpha cells of the islets of Langerhans, and insulin, which is produced from the beta cells of the islets of Langerhans. Glucagon raises blood sugar and insulin lowers blood sugar.

There are other cells within the endocrine tissue, such as delta and F cells, which produce hormones and polypeptides. These also have a role in the maintenance of glucose within the blood.

The primary problem that occurs with endocrine tissue of the pancreas causes diabetes mellitus.

Diabetes mellitus

This is a failure of the pancreas to secrete sufficient insulin to meet the body's requirements. Consequently, the blood sugar will rise (hyperglycaemia). It is a chronic disease and is common in the United Kingdom with an incidence of 2% of the population. It is more likely to occur with age and 80% of people with diabetes mellitus are over the age of 50. The cause is not understood. A family history makes it more likely that an individual will develop this problem. Other diseases of the pancreas, such as tumours and inflammation, can cause secondary diabetes, as can corticosteroid therapy.

There are three main approaches to people who have diabetes mellitus: controlling their intake of carbohydrate, controlling diet and prescribing oral drugs to lower blood sugar, and controlling diet and prescribing insulin.

Diet alone

This involves controlling the amount of carbohydrate in relation to the person's weight, occupation, age and gender. By controlling the amount of carbohydrate, and therefore glucose, one is enabling the amount of insulin that the body is producing to manage in relation to the carbodydrate being consumed.

The amount of carbohydrate will vary and must be assessed individually. The requirements will naturally not be the same for an active diabetic as opposed to an overweight, sendentary obese person.

Diet and oral drug therapy

If diet alone is not sufficient to control the blood sugar levels, then oral hypoglycaemic drugs may be required. These drugs act by reducing the release of glucose from the liver—e.g. glibenclamide, tolbutamide and chlorpropamide—or by increasing the uptake of glucose in the tissues—e.g. metformin.

Diet and insulin therapy

For some people, diet and oral hypoglycaemic drugs are not sufficient and they will therefore require insulin. Children and young people often require insulin due to the demands made on their body by growth. The person will be taught to adjust their carbohydrate intake, and also the amount of insulin they require, in relation to their individual needs.

A variety of types of insulin are available. These are chosen according to whether the person requires a short-acting, an intermediate, a long-acting, or a combination of two categories of insulin.

The role of a nurse as a health educator

The person who develops diabetes mellitus has a chronic disease with which they must live for the rest of their life. Consequently, the nurse has a critical role in ensuring that the person is knowledgeable about diabetes and how it relates to their activities of daily living. It is in the application of the knowledge they have about diabetes to leading a normal life that the nurse can have a vital role to play. In addition to providing an understanding of what diabetes mellitus is, the nurse should plan a programme of education for the person and their family in relation to the following areas.

Diet

The prescribed diet must be carefully explained. Initial instruction is normally given by a dietician and then reinforced by the nurse. The person, while in hospital, should be encouraged to select their own food for a period of time under the supervision of the nurse. Advice should be given in calculating the carbohydrate value of types of food. The information leaflets from the British Diabetic Association are particularly helpful. The importance of regular meals should be stressed. It is also important to stress the particular dangers of obesity for this group of people. If the person also requires medication, then the importance of eating in relation to the drugs being taken must be explained.

Medication

If the person is on insulin therapy then they will require education about the type and dose of insulin they require, how it works and when they require an injection. The technique of giving an injection (see Figure 14.3), the storage of insulin, the ordering of supplies, the disposal of

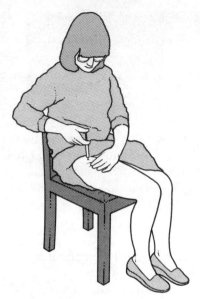

Figure 14.3 Injection of insulin.

equipment and the importance of rotating sites should be
explained.

If a person finds normal syringes difficult, then
automatic injectors, of a variety of sorts, are available.
These injectors have a mechanically controlled spring,
which, when released, pushes the needle quickly through
the skin (see Figure 14.4).

If oral hypoglycaemic drugs are prescribed then the
importance of taking the drug at the correct time, the dose
required and the side-effects of those drugs should be
explained.

Changes in lifestyle in relation to diet and drugs

People with diabetes are taught to alter their diet and
amount of medication in response to their lifestyle. This is

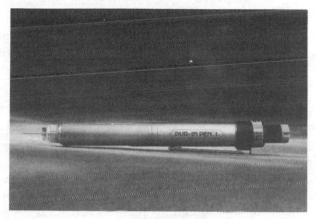

Figure 14.4 Example of an automatic injector.

of critical importance as it enables the person to lead a normal life and not be controlled by their diabetes.

If a person knows they are going to have delayed meals, or a higher than usual carbohydrate intake, or be travelling, then they will need advice on altering the time and amount of medication that they take.

It is also important that the person is aware that if they develop another illness then their requirements for insulin may be altered. Insulin requirements are also altered during pregnancy.

Assessing blood glucose levels

The importance of assessing blood glucose levels must be stressed. It is this information that enables the person to adjust their diet and medication to ensure good health. The correct technique of blood glucose monitoring should be taught. This is normally performed using BM stix, but portable machines also exist.

It is also helpful to ensure that the person understands how to assess the glucose level in their urine.

Knowledge of hypoglycaemia and hyperglycaemia

A person and their family should understand the changes that can occur when their blood sugar levels fall or rise outside the normal range. It is important that they can then take preventative measures to ensure that they do not develop a coma.

Hypoglycaemia

If blood sugar falls below normal then problems can occur rapidly. If a person recognizes that this is occurring then they should take glucose immediately. Consequently, they should always carry glucose, in a convenient form, with them. As blood sugar falls the person will first experience the following:

Trembling
Sweating
Feel nervous or restless
May describe a sense of impending doom
Act strangely and may be confused
Have clammy skin
May feel weak
May feel hungry
May have a headache
May have visual disturbances
A raised heart rate may be present but blood pressure will
    be normal

If action is not taken then clonic convulsions will occur and the person will lose consciousness. If this persists then they will become deeply comatose with shallow respirations and have a slow heart rate.

Hyperglycaemia

The problems that result with high blood glucose may develop slowly. In the first stage people may experience loss of appetite, nausea, vomiting, feelings of weakness and drowsiness. This may occur as a result of infection or stress. It is important that a person knows to seek advice if this occurs so that diet and medication can be adjusted. If these problems are not resolved and blood glucose levels continue to rise then a hyperglycaemic coma can occur.

Knowledge concerning the importance of general health, skin, foot and mouth care

People with diabetes are more prone to infection and to suffer changes to their circulatory system. They should be advised to take particular care if they do develop an infection and if it does not resolve to seek medical advice.

Foot care

The adult diabetic should take particular care of their feet due to their increased susceptibility to circulatory problems which may be compounded by a lack of sensation. Socks and shoes should fit well, feet should be dried thoroughly and toenails cut well. Many diabetics have their toenails cut by a qualified chiropodist.

Eye care

Due to vascular changes the person with diabetes is prone to retinal haemorrhage and the development of cataracts. This is important.

Support within the community

A newly diagnosed person with diabetes will need support when they leave hospital. Clinical nurse specialists in the care of people with diabetes are now based in the community. They can be of support to either the person and their family or to other community nurses involved in caring for the person. District nurses, dieticians and general practitioners are other health professionals who can help. In addition the address of the British Diabetic Association should be given to the person, together with any local support groups that exist.

Assessment of a person with diabetes mellitus

- Glycosuria—often discovered on routine urine testing.
- Polyuria due to increased osmotic pressure exerted by high concentration of glucose.
- Polydipsia—dehydration and thirst caused by polyuria.
- Weight loss, lethargy and muscle wasting. This is caused as fat is broken down for energy production instead of carbohydrate.
- Ketonuria and the smell of ketones on the breath. This occurs because ketones are the breakdown of fat metabolism.
- Nausea and vomiting due to ketoacidosis.
- Drowsiness and confusion. This can lead to a coma and death may occur.

Diabetic ketoacidosis

This condition occurs in diabetics with severe hyperglycaemia when fat is broken down for energy production. Toxic acid products of fat metabolism (ketones) accumulate in the blood. This happens with new diabetics who have not been diagnosed, or not sought medical assistance, through ignorance or carelessness, and when other illnesses and/or stress are present—this increases insulin requirements.

The assessment of their problems will largely fall within the areas that have been listed. However, they are more likely to be in a coma if their diabetes has resulted in ketone breakdown. Dehydration and electrolyte imbalance can mean that their life is threatened.

The range of problems and nursing actions required for a person with diabetes mellitus will vary according to the level of hyperglycaemia that they present with. People may require education and information about diet or may be critically ill. The problems considered below are largely concerned with a person who has diabetic ketoacidosis.

Problem

Unstable metabolic and nutritional requirements due to hyperglycaemia.

Actions

- Administer insulin as prescribed. This is normally given continuously and the amount determined by their blood sugar level.
- Assess blood sugar levels one- to two-hourly.
- Assess for signs that the person is developing hypoglycaemia. This can be caused by too rapid an administration of insulin.

Problem

Dehydration and electrolyte imbalance.

Actions

- Administer intravenous fluids and electrolytes as prescribed.
- Record fluid intake and output (the person may require catheterization if unconscious so as to record output accurately).
- Assess blood pressure and cardiac rate.
- Assess for fluid overload.

Problem

May not be able to maintain a safe environment due to altered level of consciousness.

Actions

- Ensure that airway is patent. Assess position required to nurse the person. Airway, oxygen and suction to be present.
- Assess level of consciousness (see Chapter 3).
- Assess respiratory rate, depth and distress.
- Explain all actions clearly.
- Assess the need for safety in terms of the height of the bed from the floor and position within the ward so that they are under the constant supervision of the nurses.

Problem

Anxiety and fear due to the unexpected coma and life-threatening problems.

Actions

- Assure the person about what has happened and explain that we can lessen the likelihood of it happening again through education and advice.
- Explain the nursing actions required.
- Ensure that family and friends have been contacted.

Problem

Lack of knowledge and understanding about diabetes mellitus and its problems.

Actions

- Assess knowledge of diabetes mellitus of the person and their family.
- Assess knowledge of diet, insulin, exercise, and

contributory factors such as stress or other illnesses.
- Plan a programme of teaching. Consider which other health professionals may need to be involved, e.g. clinical nurse specialist and dietician.
- Evaluate the person's and their family's understanding of the knowledge they require to lessen the risk of further problems.

THE ADRENAL GLANDS

The adrenal glands are situated on the top of each kidney and are therefore sometimes termed the suprarenal glands. Each gland consists of an outer cortex and an inner medulla.

The adrenal cortex produces glucocorticoids, mineralocorticoids and androgens. Glucocorticoids and mineralocorticoids are important in the formation of glucose, the retention of salt and water, the manufacture of red blood cells, the maintenance of blood pressure and for the response of the body to stress. Androgens help influence the development of sexual characteristics.

The adrenal cortex is controlled by the release of adrenocorticotrophic hormone (ACTH) from the anterior part of the pituitary gland.

The adrenal medulla secretes adrenaline and noradrenaline. These hormones help to prepare the body for physical exertion by increasing blood pressure, the rate at which the heart beats, and the blood supply to the muscles, brain and lungs, and by releasing glycogen for conversion to sugar.

Problems can occur from overactive or underactive adrenal glands.

Overactive adrenal glands

An overactive adrenal gland is often referred to as Cushing's syndrome. This syndrome occurs as a result of an excess of ACTH from the anterior part of the pituitary—normally caused by a tumour of the pituitary gland—or by hyperplasia of the adrenal glands. As a result an excessive secretion of hormones from the adrenal cortex occurs.

Underactive adrenal glands

An underactive adrenal gland is often referred to as Addison's disease. It is usually caused by atrophy or damage by tuberculosis of both adrenal glands. As a result an undersecretion of hormones from the adrenal cortex occurs.

Assessment

Underactive (Addison's disease)	*Overactive (Cushing's syndrome)*
Hypoglycaemia	Hyperglycaemia
Electrolyte imbalance	Electrolyte imbalance
Fluid loss and dehydration	Fluid retention and oedema
Weight loss	Weight gain
Hypotension	Hypertension
Anorexia and nausea	Muscle wasting and abnormal fat distribution
Skin can be dusky with brown pigmentation	Skin can have purple striae on buttocks and abdomen
Cardiac arrhythmias	Cardiac dysfunction
Constant fatigue and listlessness	Weakness and backache
Constipation and diarrhoea	Secondary male characteristics in females

Underactive adrenal glands may cause life-threatening problems due to electrolyte imbalance, cardiac arrhythmias and hypoglycaemia. The person will require long-term treatment with corticosteroids. The nurse has an important role to play in educating the person as to the effects, side-effects and way that these drugs work. The need to carry a steroid card at all times, and never to stop these drugs, must be stressed.

Overactive adrenal glands may also cause a range of problems. The treatment, though, is by surgery—either to the pituitary gland or to the adrenal glands themselves. The nurse's role will be to support the person through the surgery and to provide education following the surgery.

The adrenal medulla

Rare tumours can occur of the adrenal medulla. The main tumour that does occur is known as a phaeochromocytoma. This causes an overproduction of adrenaline and noradrenaline. Consequently, the person will sweat profusely, have raised blood pressure, a raised heart rate and other metabolic problems. Treatment is by the surgical removal of the tumour.

FURTHER READING

DAVIDSON, M. B. (1991). *Diabetes Mellitus: Diagnosis and Treatment*. Churchill Livingstone, London.

DILLON, R. S. (1980). *Handbook of Endocrinology*, 2nd edn. Lea and Febiger, Philadelphia.

DORNAN, T. (1988). *Diabetes Care. A Problem Solving Approach*. Heinemann Professional Publishing, Oxford.

FLETCHER, R. F. (1979). *Lecture Notes on Endocrinology*, 2nd edn. Blackwell Scientific Publications, Oxford.

LEE, J. & LAYCOCK, R. (1979). *Essential Endocrinology*. Oxford University Press, Oxford.

STEINER, G. & LAWRENCE, P. (1981). *Educating Diabetic Patients*, 2nd edn. Springer Publishing Company, London.

THOMPSON, J. A. (1981). *An Introduction to Clinical Endocrinology*, 2nd edn. Churchill Livingstone, Edinburgh.

Note: There are now specialist journals in the care of people with
    diabetes mellitus.

Diabetic Nursing, Media Medica, West Sussex.

Practical Diabetes, Maxwell Marketing Services.

15 Nursing people with problems of their bones, joints and connective tissue

The rheumatic diseases are among the commonest of all diseases. They represent one of the most important causes of suffering and economic loss from illness in any nation. Problems affecting the bones and joints are characterized by local pain, often of a persistent and chronic nature, and by varying degrees of limitation of movement and deformities. Consequently they have serious implications for the individual, their family and the community.

RHEUMATOID ARTHRITIS

Rheumatoid arthritis is a common and very crippling inflammatory disease of the joints. It is a peripheral symmetrical inflammatory disease of synovium leading to destruction of cartilage and adjacent bone, resulting in deformity and loss of function of any of the 187 synovial joints in the body. The erosions can be seen radiologically.

Although at least half a million people in Great Britain alone suffer from this painful and crippling disease, the cause is not fully understood. No single initiating factor has been isolated, although it is thought that immune overactivity plays an important role. Females are more commonly affected than males in a ratio of 3:1. Rheumatoid arthritis occurs world-wide and all age groups are affected, although the maximum incidence of onset is in the fifth decade.

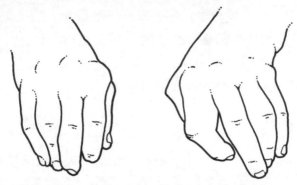

Figure 15.1   The hands of a person with rheumatoid arthritis.

Diagnosis is based on clinical examination and a history of the illness. Investigations which will help confirm the diagnosis are X-rays, screening of the blood for rheumatoid factor, erythrocyte sedimentation rate (ESR), white blood cell count, alkaline phosphatase levels, uric acid levels, and haemoglobin levels, in addition to other usual haematological tests. Occasionally fluid from an inflamed joint will be examined.

In cases of severe immobility, a replacement of a joint may be considered. Hip and knee joints are the joints most commonly replaced, but ankle and shoulder joint replacements have been performed.

The problems that a person will suffer from will vary considerably due to the extent of the disease and the particular joints involved. The onset may be insidious, with pain in one or two of the smaller joints, such as those of the fingers and toes; these may then progress and involve the wrist, elbow, shoulder, hip and knee joints. The changes lead to ankylosis (fixation of the joints) with a loss of movement (Figure 15.1). Deformity is made worse by wasting of the muscles.

In the acute phase assessment may show:

- Morning stiffness
- Tenderness or pain on movement for a period of days or weeks
- History of swelling of the joints
- Subcutaneous nodules
- Weight loss
- Loss of appetite
- Malaise and weakness
- Raised temperature

Care of a person with problems due to rheumatoid arthritis

In the absence of a cure for rheumatoid disease the care and management must be aimed at controlling the inflammatory response and preventing further structural damage.

A team approach is required, involving nurses, physicians, physiotherapists, pharmacists, dieticians, occupational therapists and social workers in full consultation with the person and their family.

The pace at which people move about and care for themselves is often slow. Consequently, ward routine needs to be adapted to this pace so that every encouragement is given to initiative and self-sufficiency.

Problem

Pain due to the inflammation of joints.

Actions

- Assess the individual's pain. This will include identifying the involved joints, the amount of swelling, redness and warmth, the range of motion of the joints and the frequency and level of pain felt.

- Bed-rest may be necessary during an acute phase of inflammation.
- Splints are applied to the inflamed joints while at rest, and later the application of functional splints may provide relief of local pain.
- The person's individual nursing should be organized so as to allow for adequate rest and exercise.
- Local injections into the joint, and the application of heat and cold, may also help.
- Administer and assess the effects of the drugs that are prescribed. (See page 368.)
- A bed cradle may be used to prevent the pressure of bed clothes on painful joints.

Problem

Potential for a person's joints to become deformed.

Actions

- Assess the mobility and functioning of the individual's joints. During the acute period of inflammation the affected joints are particularly painful on movement. The involved part usually assumes the flexed position because of the spasm of the dominant flexor muscles and contracture of the joint may occur.
- Splints may be required to reduce the severity of pain and prevent contractures and flexion deformities (see Figure 15.2). They are particularly useful for knee, wrist, elbow and finger joints. The occupational therapist and physiotherapist will help in assessing joint deformity and making the correct splint.
- A series of exercises will be used to help lessen the risk of flexion contractures. These may be passive to start with and are gradually increased to active and resistive exercises as the person's condition improves.

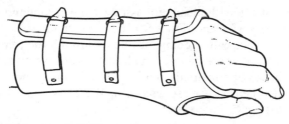

Figure 15.2 A resting splint.

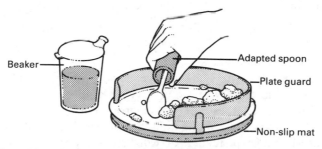

Figure 15.3 Feeding aids.

- Hot wax therapy may help with physiotherapy and exercises for deformed joints.

Problem

The person requires a well-balanced diet.

Actions

- Assess the person's weight and diet. The person requires, as all people do, a well-balanced diet. They may have weight loss and loss of appetite or may be obese. Being overweight increases the strain on joints.

- Involve the dietician in assessing nutrition and calculating a balanced diet for the individual.
- Assistance with feeding may be required if the joints of the hands or arms are involved. A variety of feeding aids can be provided such as adapted cutlery, non-stick mats, beakers, plate guards and straws (see Figure 15.3).

Problem

May have a raised temperature due to infection/inflammation.

Actions

- Assess temperature.
- Ensure that there are no secondary sources of infection, e.g. urinary or respiratory system.
- Light bed clothes and cool environment.
- If sweating is occurring then careful washing and drying and change of nightwear will help the person to feel comfortable.

Problem

May not be able to be independent due to pain and deformity of joints.

Actions

- Assess level of independence in relation to activities of daily living.
- Assistance with hygiene may be required.
- Assistance with elimination of faeces and urine may be difficult. A commode or raised lavatory seat may be easier to use than a bed pan.
- Assess risk of developing pressure sores, chest infec-

tion and deep vein thrombosis due to immobility and possible bed-rest.

Problem

The person may have a depressed mood and low self-esteem due to lack of independence, pain and disability.

Actions

- Assess the person's feelings about their health.
- Assist the person and their family in expressing their thoughts about their problems and their view of the future.
- Active listening is important.
- Identify and build on the individual's coping strategies.
- Allow time for the person and their family to express their feelings.
- Involve other disciplines so that support towards the future outside hospital is evident.

After the acute phase of problems, the person will undergo a period of remobilization. A physiotherapist is critical in guiding the person and the nursing staff in the planned programme of remobilization. This usually begins with general exercises designed to regain muscle tone and progresses to exercises to increase muscle strength and mobility of the joints. These exercises will be developed over a period of time. Hydrotherapy may aid in this programme. The nurse has an important role in supervising the exercises and providing support in ensuring that the programme is followed correctly.

The next phase of the care of a person with rheumatoid arthritis is concerned with rehabilitation. During this period the person is independent within the limits of their disease. The person should be encouraged to wear their own clothes and to go to the day room for meals. The nurse should assess the need for social workers, disablement resettlement officers and community nurses in relation to the person and their family life at home. A home assessment by the physiotherapist, occupational therapist, social worker and nurse may be necessary.

During this phase the nurse must ensure that the person understands about their ill-health and the care they require outside hospital. The nurse should assess the person's knowledge, and plan and evaluate a programme of education. The areas of knowledge that they should consider involve:

- Drug therapy. The effects and side-effects of the drugs that the person is taking should be understood. They may be on some of their drugs for the remainder of their lives and so must know why they are on those drugs, the dose to be taken, when to take that drug, how to obtain further supplies and the side-effects that may occur as a result of taking those drugs (see Drug therapy).
- Nutrition. The person and their family should understand how to continue to take a balanced diet and a dietician will help with this information.
- The person should understand the exercises that they should continue, the use of any aids to living that have been provided and the importance of maintaining a good body alignment.
- Follow-up support. The person should understand the follow-up nursing and medical support that is needed. Information leaflets from the Arthritis Research Council and addresses of national and local support organizations should be given.

Drug therapy

Drug therapy is widely used for people with problems resulting from rheumatoid arthritis. People and those caring for them need to understand the actions and problems involved in giving these drugs. People may stay on drug treatment for the remainder of their lives. Where possible, self-medication of drugs should be practised in hospital prior to a person going home. This enables nurses to assess a person's knowledge and understanding of their drug therapy.

Some of the drugs prescribed are as follows.

Non-steroidal anti-inflammatory drugs

Acetylsalicylic acid (aspirin) is commonly used. It may be prescribed in relatively large doses. This can cause gastrointestinal disturbances, ringing in the ears and general problems of hearing. It may be helpful to give this drug in enteric form and it should be given with, or just after, food.

Ibuprofen (Brufen) and indomethacin (Indocid) are two other common non-steroidal anti-inflammatory drugs. Both may cause gastrointestinal problems, with nausea and vomiting being prominent. Other drugs within this group that can be used are naproxen (Naprosyn) and fenoprofen (Fenopron).

Adrenal corticosteroids

This group of drugs, such as prednisolone and hydro-cortisone, is used for people when their inflammatory process is severe or rapidly progressing. It may be given for a particular period of time and the dose may be altered over a course of treatment. These forms of steroid drugs are powerful and the person needs to understand the range of problems that can occur, the need not to stop these drugs, and the importance of carrying a steroid card, in addition to the dose and when and how to take them.

D-Penicillamine

This is an oral anti-inflammatory drug. It works over a period of months and so benefits are not immediately apparent. It is used for people who have severe rheumatoid arthritis which may not have responded to other drugs. Its side-effects include anorexia, nausea, vomiting, thrombocytopenia and renal damage.

Gold compounds

A preparation of gold salts such as sodium aurothiamalate (Myocrisin) may be given, often in combination with a non-steroidal drug. This is normally given by intramuscular injection over a period of three to six months. People need to be observed closely for signs of a toxic reaction. People can develop skin damage, renal damage and changes in their bone marrow which lead to severe anaemia, leucopenia and thrombocytopenia. As a result they have regular assessment of their urine and blood count.

Other groups of drugs that can be used include antimalarial and immunosuppressive drugs. These can cause severe side-effects and so the person and the nursing staff must be aware of these.

OSTEOARTHROSIS

Osteoarthrosis is a disease in which pathological wear in joints occurs. Advancing age is accompanied by degenerative changes affecting all the tissues of the body to a varying extent. Osteoarthrosis or degenerative joint disease represents the degenerative process affecting the joints. The term osteoarthrosis is preferred to the term osteoarthritis, as the latter term implies that there is an inflammatory basis for the condition. Osteoarthrosis is a common form of joint disease, particularly in older people.

There are two types of osteoarthrosis—primary and secondary. Primary osteoarthrosis involves many joints and is described as idiopathic, i.e. the cause is unknown. Secondary osteoarthrosis frequently involves only one joint and there is an obvious predisposing cause, e.g. a previous fracture.

Assessment

Pain in affected joint(s)
– two types of pain
    venous (constant deep ache)
    ligamentous (sharp pain on weight bearing)
Progressive loss of movement in joint
Swelling and redness of joint

In contrast to rheumatoid arthritis, this is a disease of the joints alone rather than a general disease. The pain is not caused by inflammation, so pain relief is often given by drugs which are only analgesics rather than those which are also anti-inflammatory drugs.

Physiotherapy is often helpful in alleviating pain in the joint and, more particularly, for strengthening the joint and increasing the degree of mobility. Hydrotherapy is sometimes beneficial as the warmth of the water helps to relax the muscle spasm and the buoyancy reduces the weight borne by the joint, so allowing greater movement.

Diet is only important if the patient is obese, as this will put unnecessary strain on weight-bearing joints. In such cases an appropriate reducing diet will be started.

In cases where immobility is severe, surgery will be considered.

INFECTIONS

Some people experience arthralgia (aching in the joints) or myalgia (aching in the muscles) during the course of an infection. Occasionally musculoskeletal symptoms form part of an infectious disease and, rarely, the joint itself may be the site of an infection.

Infection within a joint is a very serious condition as it can destroy the joint and may be life-threatening. Pyogenic organisms, tuberculosis and brucella can cause infection of the joints. Diagnosis is made by aspirating fluid from the joint for microbiological examination. Once an organism has been isolated, an appropriate antibiotic will be prescribed. Most antibiotics can be given systemically as they penetrate into the synovial fluid, but occasionally local administration of an antibiotic will be required.

Some infections give rise to a reactive synovitis, although infection is not present in the joint. Such diseases include brucellosis, Reiter's disease, syphilis and gonorrhoea.

Viral infections

Aching of joints and muscles is usually due to a virus infection, and the aching subsides with the fever. Viral infections such as rubella (German measles) or mumps may cause synovitis.

GOUT

Gout is caused by an accumulation of excess amounts of uric acid in the body. Uric acid is produced mainly from breakdown of nucleic acids which are found in the nuclei of cells. Some uric acid is therefore normally found in the blood and urine. High levels of uric acid in the blood may be due to one of the following mechanisms: there may be an over-production of uric acid; there may be under-excretion of uric acid by the kidney; or there may be a combination of these two. Surgery has been known to provoke an acute attack of gout.

Assessment

Pain in the affected joint
– commonly the metatarsophalangeal joint of the big toe
– sudden onset
– excruciating pain
– redness and swelling
Temperature may be raised
Nausea and vomiting may be present

Problem

Pain.

Actions

- Assess level of pain.
- Give prescribed drugs and monitor and report their effectiveness. The main drugs that are used are anti-inflammatory drugs such as indomethacin and phenyl-butazone. In addition, allopurinal may be used. This interferes with the formation of uric acid by inhibiting the enzyme xanthine oxidase.
- If the person is in bed ensure that a bed cradle is used, as even the pressure of light bed clothes causes excruciating pain.

Problem

Potential to form urate crystals in the kidney.

Actions

- Ensure high fluid intake of three litres in 24 hours. This will help to prevent the formation of crystals.
- Assess and record fluid intake and output.

Problem

Lack of knowledge about diet.

Actions

Involve dietician in advice about diet. This is controversial. However, people are normally advised to moderate their alcohol intake and refrain from high-purine foods such as liver, kidneys, beans and peas.

ANKYLOSING SPONDYLITIS

Ankylosing spondylitis is a progressive inflammatory disease affecting predominantly young males. It is characterized by spinal rigidity and limitation of chest expansion. Its cause is unknown. Unlike rheumatoid arthritis, it affects both the synovial and cartilagenous joints.

Assessment

Pain and stiffness in lower part of back
- unrelieved by rest
- worse in the morning
Chest pain
- due to involvement of costo-vertebral joints (where ribs join spine)
Rigidity of chest movement
- chest expansion is limited

- breathing is usually diaphragmatic (causing abdominal bulging or ballooning)

Anorexia

Loss of weight

Synovitis

Iritis

Postural changes

- lumbar spine flattened
- upper thoracic spine bent
- neck craned forward
- chest flattened
- known as 'Bechterer stoop' or 'hang dog' appearance
- fusion of spine can result causing a rigid 'poker back'

Problem

Pain.

Actions

- Assess level, type and severity of pain.
- Assess effectiveness of any drugs prescribed. Analgesia is sometimes prescribed in the acute period, such as aspirin. In addition, anti-inflammatory drugs may be used, such as indomethacin, naproxen and phenylbutazone.
- Assess whether heat, cold or massage help with the pain.

Problem

Potential to develop deformities related to posture.

Actions

- Mobilization is vital. People are encouraged to exercise in order to prevent postural abnormality and limitation of movement of the spine, chest and peripheral joints.

- Involvement of the physiotherapist is important to instruct the person and the nursing staff on the appropriate exercises. These should be continued when the person leaves hospital.
- Hydrotherapy may be beneficial and swimming should be encouraged.
- The person should lie on a firm bed with a supportive mattress.

Problem

Anxiety over future changes which may occur.

Actions

- Ensure that all information is shared with the person and their family. As the future is unsure it is important that people feel involved with their care.
- Ensure that information is clearly and well explained.

Problem

Potential for poor nutrition and weight loss.

Actions

- Assess nutritional status and weight.
- Involve dietician to assess nutrition and plan an adequate nutritional intake.
- Weigh twice weekly.
- Assess the person's understanding of their future nutritional requirements.

Problem

Need for education and advice.

Actions

- Assess knowledge and understanding.
- Plan a programme of education to include consideration of: type of exercises to be performed; effects and
  side-effects of any drugs; need for nutrition and the
  follow-up support that has been planned.

If the disease is progressing and there is concern about the
development of severe iritis then corticosteroids may be
considered. This is rare. If this form of drug therapy is
required then education about the use, dosage, and side-
effects of these drugs will be necessary.

RHEUMATIC FEVER

Rheumatic fever or acute rheumatism is mainly a disease
of children and young adults. It is associated with
haemolytic streptococcal infections. However, it is not
direct infection by these organisms which causes the
disease, but a probable abnormality in the body's immune
response to the invading streptococci. The streptococci
may have originally caused a mild infection, such as a sore
throat, and then, due to the possible abnormality of the
immune system's response, go on to cause acute rheumatic fever and rheumatic heart disease. Improvement in
social conditions and the use of penicillin has meant that
the incidence of this disease is declining.

The main features of this disease are polyarthritis,
chorea and carditis, of which carditis is the most important
as it may cause permanent damage to the heart.

Assessment

Fever
– usually 38–39°C
– may be higher

Joint pains
– many joints involved for short periods
– pain moves from joint to joint
– joints are hot, red, tender and swollen
Subcutaneous nodules
– vary in size
– may be large swellings
– may be barely palpable
Skin rash
– on trunk and limbs
Malaise
Lethargy
Anorexia
Weakness
Cardiac damage
Chorea
– involuntary muscular spasm
– usually involves face and hands
– emotional lability
– also known as St Vitus' dance

Problem

Raised temperature due to infection.

Actions

- Assess and record temperature. This may be raised to 38–39°C, although it can be higher.
- Aspirin 1–2 g four-hourly may be required to bring the temperature down. These high doses of aspirin may cause nausea, headaches, deafness and ringing in the ears. Any of these problems should be reported.
- Fanning and tepid sponging may be necessary.
- A high fluid intake is maintained to lower the

temperature and to prevent dehydration which may have been caused by profuse sweating.

- Washing and drying of the skin and a change of nightwear is required after a sweating attack to aid the person's comfort.
- Penicillin may be prescribed. It does not directly affect the inflammation of the joints but combats the primary cause of the infection, e.g. streptococcal infection of the tonsils.

Problem

Potential for cardiac damage.

Actions

- Bed-rest may be required in the initial phase to lessen the risk of cardiac damage. This is assessed individually and is now rarely as long as it used to be, when six weeks on bed-rest was not uncommon.
- An electrocardiograph (ECG) will be performed to assess whether cardiac damage is present.
- Blood pressure and cardiac rate will be assessed.
- Corticosteroids such as prednisolone may be used to lessen the risk of heart valves becoming thickened and deformed. The damage to the valves of the heart is of particular concern.

Problem

Potential for joint deformity.

Actions

- Involve the physiotherapist with advice on appropriate exercises.

- Light splints may be helpful.
- A bed cradle may also be necessary.

Problem

Anxiety over the future.

Actions

- Ensure that explanations are clear and that all information is shared with the person.
- If the person is to remain in hospital for a long period of time there may be financial consequences and a social worker should be involved.

If, although it is now rare, prolonged bed-rest is necessary, then assessment of the risks of remaining in bed and the person's activities of daily living should take place.

DIFFUSE CONNECTIVE TISSUE DISEASE

This group of diseases, formerly called collagen diseases, may affect the connective tissue throughout the body. Their effects are widespread, and the involvement of many different systems of the body means they are encountered in both medicine and surgery. In addition to the two diseases described, there are three other main diffuse connective tissue diseases: systemic sclerosis, polymyositis and dermatomyositis.

Systemic lupus erythematosus (SLE)

This is a diffuse disorder of connective tissue associated with vasculitis. It has a variety of manifestations. It commonly presents with arthralgia, fever, malaise and weight loss. A rash often occurs on the face. Pleural and pericardial effusions are frequent, and atelectasis (collapse) may occur at the lung bases.

Involvement of the kidneys occurs in about one third of cases. In addition, central nervous system involvement is being recognized more frequently. The cause is unknown.

Diagnosis of this disease may be difficult. It is based on the clinical picture and a series of haematological investigations.

Treatment consists mainly of drug therapy. Corticosteroids are the main drugs used. Analgesic and anti-inflammatory drugs may be given for the joint pain. Avoidance of sunlight and the use of corticosteroid cream may help the facial skin rash.

Unless there is involvement of the renal system, the prognosis is improving steadily as treatment becomes more effective.

Polyarteritis nodosa (PAN)

This disease involves the inflammation of the medium-sized and small arteries and is characterized by segmental vessel wall necrosis. Arteries throughout the body may be involved. The cause is unknown. Polyarteritis nodosa occurs more commonly in males than females and, although it may start at any age, it is most common in young adults.

The features of the illness are widespread. A person will present with malaise, weakness, pyrexia and weight loss. Peripheral neuropathy, heart failure, alterations in gastrointestinal function, joint pain and kidney involvement may occur. This latter problem may lead to hypertension and renal failure. Diagnosis is made by examination of a biopsy of the affected part; muscle or kidney biopsies are commonly used.

Treatment is normally with high-dose corticosteroids; doses of 60 mg/day may be given.

FURTHER READING

BLUESTONE, R. (ed.) (1980). *Rheumatology*, 2nd edn. Lea and Febiger, Philadelphia.

ELLIOTT, M. (1979). *Nursing Rheumatic Disease*. Churchill Livingstone, Edinburgh.

GRENNAN, D. M. (1984). *Rheumatology*. Baillière Tindall, London.

LAARIK, K., LAURIN, J. & GINES, G. E. S. (1984). Arthritis self-management: a five year history of a patient education program. *Nursing Clinics of North America*, **1**, No. 4, 637–645.

MOONEY, N. (1983). Coping with chronic pain in rheumatoid arthritis: patient behaviour and nursing interventions. *Rehabilitation Nursing*, **8**, No. 2, 20–25.

MOSKOWITZ, R. W. (1982). *Clinical Rheumatology*, 2nd edn. Lea and Febiger, Philadelphia.

PANAYI, G. S. (1980). *Essential Rheumatology for Nurses and Therapists*. Baillière Tindall, London.

PIGG, J. S., DRISCOLL, P. W. & CANIFF, R. (1985). *Rheumatology Nursing: Problem Solving Approach*. Wiley Medical Publications, Chichester.

STRAUSS, A. L. *et al.* (eds) (1984). *Chronic Illness and Quality of Life*, 2nd edn. C.V. Mosby, St Louis.

Index